I0791079

**How To Win Your War Against Bronchitis**



# Read all my books on Kindle for free without downloading and printing except you want to buy.

# Contents

# The Causes Of Bronchitis

Bronchitis is a condition in which you can have an illness that is both infectious and one that is noninfectious. In most cases, it is a virus that causes bronchitis to happen. This virus is generally the same type that causes a common cold to happen in most people.

On the other hand, bronchitis can also be a condition that is caused by the pollutants in the air that you breathe including from cigarette smoke. Smog and chemicals that are used to clean with are additional causes for bronchitis.

Another cause of bronchitis happens because of the acids that are normally found in your stomach backing up, literally, up into your gastro esophageal track. This is sometimes called GERD, or gastro esophageal reflux disease.

Some people that work in conditions that are not favorable for good, clean breathing also develop bronchitis. This type of bronchitis is known as an occupational bronchitis in which case the pollutants including dusts and/or fumes get into the breathing airways and cause illness.

Usually, when the person stops working there, or improves the breathing circumstances, their bronchitis symptoms also improve and often the irritation will stop.

The causes of chronic bronchitis are often a bit more drastic. If you have this condition, the walls of your bronchial tubes have become thickened and they are inflamed to such a degree that it is considered nearly permanent. When this happens, chronic bronchitis is evident.

Most with this condition must cough at least some time during each day to clear their throat. This is especially true of those that have chronic bronchitis due to their smoking habits. If you have to cough at least one time every day for at least three months of the year, you are considered to have chronic bronchitis.

Chronic bronchitis is often caused by smoking, but it's not the only time that you can get it. You can also get chronic bronchitis from air pollution that is severe or toxic gasses that are in the area in which you work.

**How To Win Your War Against Bronchitis**

Those that suffer from chronic symptoms of bronchitis often develop asthma because of it. This is caused by the long term inflammation of your air passageways. In any case, it is essential that you get help from your doctor in dealing with your condition. Those that are suffering from chronic bronchitis have a very serious illness to consider.

# Seeking A Doctor's Help For Bronchitis

Depending on the type of bronchitis that you have and its severity determines if you should seek help from a doctor for it. We've talked about when you need to seek a doctor's help in the last chapter. But, what happens when you go to visit your doctor?

To determine if you have bronchitis, your doctor will likely listen to your chest. This helps him to determine what is happening inside by listening for mucus build ups. In addition, he or she may also do a chest x-ray which will show the inflamed and enlarged air passageways that are likely the problem.

Some doctors will also want a sample of the mucus to determine what type and how much bacteria are in your system. The sample will consider the amount of bacteria found in the sputum when you cough.

Those that are suffering from chronic bronchitis are likely to have additional testing to insure that that is what you are suffering from.

The doctor will do a series of tests that will take into account your symptoms for conditions such as asthma and emphysema. To do this, a pulmonary function test which is also called a PFT will be used. During this test, you are told to blow into a device which is called a spirometer. This determines how much volume of air your lungs have after you take a deep breath and have blown it out.

The test is simple and takes just a minute to perform. It causes you no pain at all. In fact, if you have had bronchitis several times in the past year, ask your doctor to perform a pulmonary function test to help to determine if there is a possibility of facing chronic bronchitis.

Generally, from these tests, your doctor will be able to rule bronchitis or not. If you are diagnosised with it, the next step will be to treat it, and if treatment is even needed in your case. Doctors will determine the level of severity as well as the likeliness of treatment that you need.

If your doctor determines that you have asthma, or that your chronic condition is likely to develop asthma, then he or she may recommend additional treatment for your condition. Those

**How To Win Your War Against Bronchitis**

that are diagnosised with asthma will need an inhaler and sometimes additional asthma medications.

These products have the goal of reducing the amount of inflammation in your air passageways as well as open them up to allow for better passage to your lungs. This type of medication can be vitally important to those suffering from asthma.

From looking at your test results and listening to your lungs, your doctor will determine the right type of treatment for your condition. Usually in cases of acute conditions, this treatment is simply rest and fluids.

Yet, in the cases of chronic conditions, it is all the more important to provide you with the help you need through additional medication. Without this medication, your condition can worsen into a life threatening condition such as pneumonia.

# What Can Happen If You Don't Get Treatment

Although for most people bronchitis does not lead to anything more than a few days in bed and perhaps a bit of weight loss, for some it can lead to problems and complications that can span a lifetime.

Acute bronchitis is the least likely to do this. This is the type of bronchitis that follows a cold or other respiratory condition and usually requires very little to not prescription medication or even a doctor's visit. Yet, this is not the only type that should be considered.

In some people who are more prone to difficulties from illnesses, one single case of bronchitis, even acute bronchitis can lead to complications. For example, in some older people, this type of bronchitis can lead to pneumonia.

Those that have additional health concerns such as those that are smokers can also get to this point. In addition, infants and the elderly have naturally weaker immune systems and they too are more likely to experience problems with complications.

In these cases, individuals will need to seek medical attention so that the bronchitis can be monitored as well as treated with any type of medication that can be used. In those that have severe cases, hospitalization may be required to help.

For some individuals, bronchitis happens often. This is what is called chronic bronchitis. In these individuals, the bronchitis may not go away, but may lessen in its severity. When this happens, individuals need to be aware of it and seek the help that's needed as soon as possible.

Chronic bronchitis is a serious health condition that can lead to or even tell you that there is something else wrong with the body.

For example, chronic bronchitis can be an indication that you are suffering from asthma or lung disorders. In fact, those that do suffer from chronic bronchitis are more likely to end up with lung cancer than those that do not. Lung cancer is one of the leader's in death among people that smoke for long periods of time.

**How To Win Your War Against Bronchitis**

Remember that you don't have to smoke yourself to be a victim of what smoke can do. Just being exposed to it over long periods of time puts you at risk.

Chronic bronchitis is also a condition which affects your quality of life. You can't do the things that you like to do without suffering from breathlessness. You cough all of the time and your chest hurts. You are sick to more extreme levels when a cold just brushes by others.

These things can cause you to feel sick all of the time. That lessens your quality of life and makes you emotionally drained at the same time. Although this is only an additional part of the condition to deal with, it still bothers people enough to make a difference.

# Chronic Bronchitis And Emphysema

If you are suffering from chronic bronchitis and/or emphysema, acute bronchitis seems like nothing more than a cold. This condition is one in which severity is a serious issue for your well being.

Chronic bronchitis is a lung disease. It, along with emphysema, is known as COPD, or chronic obstructive pulmonary disease. This condition is one that refers to the obstruction of the air passageways that stops you from breathing normally. You can have both emphysema and chronic bronchitis at the same time. Here are some facts you should know about chronic bronchitis.

1. COPD claims some 122,000 deaths each year in the US, as claimed by a study done in 2003. It is one of the leading causes of death.

2. The largest risk factor in patients that get COPD is that of smoking. 80 to 90 percent of those that suffer from this condition will be smokers. 90 percent of them will die from it because they smoked.

3. Female smokers are more likely to get COPD than men are.

4. If you are a victim of air pollution, second hand smoke, or have a history of infections of the respiratory system, you have an increased risk of getting COPD.

5. 19 percent of those that suffer from COPD will get it from their work environment.

It is estimated that some 11 million people in the United States alone have chronic bronchitis or emphysema yet many more are believed to suffer from it but are under diagnosised by it. In the population of aged Americans, of a frightening 700,000 hospital discharges, 70 percent of them were in people that are over the age of 65 (in 2004) showing the real risk that this condition poses to those that are older.

## How To Win Your War Against Bronchitis

Those that suffer from chronic bronchitis start by having an inflammation of their bronchial tubes. These are your air passageways, remember and therefore are very important to be clear so that air can move easily in and out of them allowing you to breathe.

During your initial bouts of chronic bronchitis, your symptoms are the same as those that a person with acute bronchitis will face. There is a heavy discharge of mucus from your coughing and the cough itself is a tell tale sign of chronic bronchitis.

One thing that your doctor's will determine is if there is something else wrong that could possibly be causing your bronchitis in the first place. Some will have additional conditions like asthma that can lead to this problem. But, when there are no underlying causes, bronchitis can be labeled as the cause of your illness and then treated as such.

When you have a bronchitis bout, your bronchial tubes become inflamed and swollen. Each time that this happens, the lining of those tubes becomes scarred. Over time, the more irritation that happens the more excessive mucus production will become. Your tubes lining will become thickened because of the scarring.

As this happens, your cough becomes more and more troublesome. The excessive mucus and the scaring lead to problems with air flow. You can't breathe as easily as you did. Still, the progression worsens so that your lungs become scarred themselves.

# The Lifestyle Changes That Are Necessary

If you are suffering from chronic bronchitis, there are necessary lifestyle changes that will in fact save your life. If you plan to continue to worsen, keep doing what you are doing now. If you want to improve your health, you have to make very important yet very difficult decisions. There's no easy way around it. Unfortunately, giving up some of your freedoms will improve your chances of surviving what chronic bronchitis will do to you.

Through a few changes in your lifestyle, you will increase your longevity. You will not add a more punishment to the condition that you are already facing. What's more is that you give your body the chance to improve some of the damage that's been done to you.

You knew we were going to say it, but smoking is the cause of your chronic bronchitis and therefore you simply must stop doing it. This is the hardest part of the process of improving your lifestyle in the hopes of prolonging your life.

If you continue to smoke, you continue to add damage to your lungs and your bronchial tubes, worsening your condition, pushing you farther and faster through the stages of chronic bronchitis and ultimately shutting off your oxygen supply completely.

If you stop smoking, you stop adding additional damage to your lungs. You slow the progression of the disease significantly and, in some case, your body can repair some of the damage that has been done. Although the most difficult decision that you have to make, it is the one that will have the most significant difference in the life of a person suffering from chronic bronchitis.

The good news is that there is quite a bit of help to the smoker today that can aid them in improving their chances of stopping this habit.

Smoking, including that of cigarette smoke and even marijuana smoking damages the lungs and is one of the general causes of chronic bronchitis.

If you work in an area that the air quality is poor, then you need to improve this quality or stop working there. Chronic bronchitis can be brought on by the air that you breathe if it is not as clean as it should be.

**How To Win Your War Against Bronchitis**


Chemicals in the air as well as pollutants can do the same damage as smoking does. Therefore, you need to take into consideration the need for improvement of the air quality that you breathe.

If the air that you breathe is not healthy, then improvement is necessary. Remove contaminants that are in the air. Reduce the use of chemicals that can also cause pollution. If this is your work environment, speak to your supervisor about moving to a more clean air area. In addition, contact your human resource manager about your rights for clean air in the work place.

# Acute Bronchitis: Knowing About The Different Signs And Symptoms

Many people suffer from a variety of respiratory disorders. It is important that your respiratory system remains in a healthy condition. Many people ignore the early signs of a respiratory disorder, as a result of which they are unable to control a condition that can later becomes chronic and lead to disability. For example, acute bronchitis, when neglected, leads to chronic bronchitis, a condition that causes severe, irreversible damage to your respiratory system and leaves you disabled for life. Therefore, updating your knowledge about bronchitis and its various signs and symptoms is of utmost importance. Neglect of this condition could lead to a medical as well as a personal disaster.

## What is Acute Bronchitis?

Acute bronchitis is a disease of the respiratory system caused due to viral infection of the bronchial tree. In some cases, the infecting agent is a fungus. Usually, people mistake this condition to be common cold and underestimate the seriousness of it. This is the common reason why most people tend to ignore bronchitis.

Children and infants are easy prey for this condition because their immune systems are still in the growing phase and are not that well-equipped to battle the virus. Bronchitis also affects tobacco smokers and those who reside in highly polluted cities.

## Treatment for Bronchitis

If the condition is acute bronchitis caused by a virus, it does not require any special treatment. All that you need to do is rest and relax as much as possible and drink plenty of fluids such as water and the juices of fruits and vegetables. If you or someone at home is suffering from bronchitis, it is highly advisable that you use humidifiers to raise the humidity in the rooms. If this is not possible, place wet towels or blankets in different areas of the house. A humid condition is ideal for the recovery of a person suffering from bronchitis.

Acute bronchitis does not last more than 10-12 days if treated properly. Usually, it is closely followed by a flue or cold. You might also cough for 2-3 weeks, and you will continue to cough till your bronchioles are completely healed and free of infection. If the cough persists, it may be due to another condition. In this case, you need to consult your physician and get yourself checked for any other medical condition. It is very important to know that acute bronchitis, if left unattended to, can lead to a condition called chronic bronchitis. This can cause intense misery and last from 3 months to two years. Moreover, it can permanently damage your respiratory system.

## Signs and Symptoms of Bronchitis

You know that you are in for acute bronchitis when you experience breathlessness, slight pain and tightness in the chest, light fever, chills, persistent cough that brings out a lot of mucus, wheezing, and headache. Now, this can easily be mistaken for a common cold. Only a doctor can make out the difference. So, as soon as you experience these symptoms, visit your family doctor and get a medical examination.

A number of tests are required to determine if you are suffering from acute bronchitis or just a common cold. A doctor will study your breathing pattern through a stethoscope. Chest X-rays will be taken. Laboratory tests will be conducted to examine your mucus in order to determine if the condition has been caused by bacteria, virus, or fungus.

## Recovering from Bronchitis

If you are diagnosed with acute bronchitis, quit smoking immediately. Avoid cigarette smoke completely if you want a speedy recovery. Smoke is really bad for you, so is polluted air. Ensure than the air around you is perfectly clean. You can do so by installing an air purifier or two inside your house.

## Prevention of Acute Bronchitis

You don't need to suffer from acute bronchitis. You can easily prevent it by taking a few precautions. It is important to avoid getting infected by virus, bacteria, and fungi that cause acute bronchitis, and you can do so by washing your hands regularly and giving up smoking.

**How To Win Your War Against Bronchitis**

Never ever ignore the signs of acute bronchitis. Visit your doctor to ascertain once and for all if what you have caught is acute bronchitis or just a common cold. Don't take the decision yourself.

The health of your respiratory system is in your control. Keep yourself informed about acute bronchitis and understand its symptoms well. You can prevent it from turning into a chronic condition simply by taking the right treatment at the right time.

# <u>Allergic Bronchitis: Understanding This Illness And Ways To Treat It</u>

Millions of Americans suffer from one respiratory disorder or the other, which can impact their lives in serious ways. A respiratory disorder can be acute or chronic. Acute disorders can be easily treated and last for a short time. On the other hand, chronic disorders are not only difficult to treat but can also leave a person disabled for life.

## What is Allergic Bronchitis?

Allergic bronchitis is a type of respiratory disorder. It is commonly referred to as allergic asthma. The immune system of a person suffering from allergic bronchitis is highly sensitive and so hyperactive that it attacks even harmless foreign substance that enters the body. To put it in other words, the immune system labels a harmless entrant into the body as "dangerous" and produces antibodies to fight against it.

In allergic bronchitis, irritants and allergens inflame the bronchi and lower parts of the respiratory system. The condition lasts as long as the person is exposed to the allergens. In addition, allergic bronchitis is closely associated with asthma and respiratory allergy and can lead to conditions such as hay fever and allergic rhinitis.

In most cases, allergic bronchitis causes mild to moderate suffering. However, it is important to realize that allergic bronchitis can become very dangerous and even cause death. This is because some people are extremely sensitive to allergens. This extreme sensitivity can lead to suffocation caused due to the blocking of airways by inflamed tissues. People in this condition are in great danger. They need immediate hospitalization and medical care.

You know you are a victim of allergic bronchitis when you suffer from breathlessness, runny nose, red or swollen eyes, hyperventilation, tight chest, tickling in throat, persistent sneezing or coughing, headache, nausea, and so on. As soon as you recognize these symptoms, seek the help of a medical practitioner.

# Treatment Of Allergic Bronchitis

The importance of consulting a physician as soon you notice symptoms of allergic bronchitis cannot be overstressed. The doctor will conduct the required steps to find out which type of allergen is responsible for your particular problem. The test involves injecting an allergen directly under the skin and observing the way your body reacts to it.

Your doctor might even ask you to see an allergist. Allergists perform a series of tests in order to understand the nature of your allergy to a particular allergen. In addition, allergists can also teach you how to prevent the relapse of allergic bronchitis.

Treating mild or moderate allergic bronchitis is fairly simple. You need plenty of knowledge about the disorder, and you also need to know the particular type of allergen responsible for your problem. Once you know, it is easy to just avoid the allergens responsible for your problem. The medical treatment for this condition is anti-histamine medication.

## Prevention of Allergic Bronchitis

It is easy to manage and even prevent allergic bronchitis. As mentioned previously, the easiest way is to determine the particular allergen causing your problem and just stay away from it. In addition to this, it pays to know a few things such as the following.

The summer season can aggravate this condition simply because during the summer, there are plenty of allergens in the air.

Remember to bathe your pets regularly and free their fur from any allergens. A lot of allergens are frequently found in the fur of animals.

Take special care of yourself if you are suffering from allergic bronchitis. As already said, the condition can get dangerous.

Keep some anti-histamine medication with you while travelling. You never know the type of allergens you might come across in an unfamiliar location. Having some anti-histamine with you will help you easily control any allergic reaction that might come up.

**How To Win Your War Against Bronchitis**


Be assured that it is possible to live a full, happy, and productive life even with allergic bronchitis. It is very important to keep yourself informed about your condition, ways of treating it, and way of preventing it. Be in touch with your allergist and your doctor. They are the best people to give you all the information you require about allergic bronchitis and to teach you how to live with the problem effectively.

# Dealing With Medical Disorders

Age can weaken the various systems of your body and leave you susceptible to a wide range of maladies. However, you can prevent the occurrence of these disorders with proper life management. Here are some tips to help you deal with health conditions such as arthritis, asthma, chronic bronchitis, diabetes, heart disease, and emphysema

## Arthritis

Age and climatic conditions are the main factors responsible for this disorder. It is characterized by lack of lubricating fluids in the joints, which raises friction between the joints, cartilages, and joint linings and causes excruciating pain. The joints of a person with arthritis not only irritate but also become stiff. Continuous movement can lead to inflammation and pain.

There are two types of arthritis: osteoarthritis and rheumatoid arthritis. In osteoarthritis, the lack of lubricant causes excessive friction in the cartilage. In rheumatoid arthritis, the same happens with the joint lining.

You can deal with arthritis better by improving your knowledge about it. Often, knowledge about a disorder indicates its cure. If you are suffering from arthritis, you need a lot of oil rich in omega 3, a substance that your body cannot produce on its own. You have to receive it through proper diet. Some of the omega 3 rich sources are fish, nuts, and vegetables. The polysaturated fats found in vegetables and fish are an excellent cure for arthritis.

## Asthma

You can deal with asthma, a respiratory disorder that causes havoc with your breathing, by simply correcting defective breathing patterns. Perform certain breathing exercises involving patterns of inhalation and exhalation to control this disease. Major lifestyle changes with regard to exercise and diet are also necessary. In addition to breathing exercises, eat plenty of green leafy vegetables, fresh fruits, and roots. It is important to make special note of the fact that animal-based foods, processed foods, and grains aggravate asthma and worsen your condition.

How To Win Your War Against Bronchitis

This breathing exercise will help you manage and control asthma. While performing it, lie flat or sit erect. If the time taken by you to inhale is four seconds, the ratio of inhalation to exhalation must be 1:2. Gradually increase the time you take to inhale and exhale till your breathing pattern returns to normal. Next, concentrate on breath retention. Before exhaling, hold your breath for sometime. If the time you take to inhale is four seconds, the ratio of inhalation, retention, and exhalation should be 1:4:2.

## Chronic Bronchitis

Cigarette smokers and people with a weak immune system normally fall prey to this disorder. It can be caused by either virus or bacteria and can lead to pneumonia.

If you ever find yourself a victim of chronic bronchitis, you need to treat it continuously till it is completely cured; otherwise, you might have a relapse. Decongestants are commonly taken in order to treat this disorder.

## Diabetes

The level of blood sugar in case of diabetics is abnormally high. The chief cause of diabetes is the body's inability to produce insulin or a defect in the way insulin acts. In some cases, it is both. Diabetes is a serious medical condition, which has to be taken seriously and cannot be neglected or ignored.

To determine if you have diabetes, your physician will check the amount of sugar present in your blood; this is your blood glucose level. If you have been diagnosed with the disease, it is time to approach a dietician because you need to make major dietary changes. A dietician will help you make an effective meal plan that won't send your blood sugar level shooting up. Diabetes also means that you need to take a lot of medicines in order to control your blood sugar level. These medicines must be taken as per your doctor's instructions.

## Heart Disease

Heart disease, considered to be the number one killer in American, kills around 1.2 million Americans annually. Unfortunately, about a quarter of the Americans don't even know that they are suffering from some form of heart disease or the other. To prevent heart diseases or to entirely eliminate the risk of heart disease, you need to make major changes in your lifestyle. Simple things such as regular exercise and a healthy diet that includes nutritional supplements that are good for the heart should be incorporated into day-to-day life. In addition, you must quit smoking if you are a smoker, give up alcohol if you are hard drinker, and say no to fatty foods if you want to have a healthy heart.

## Emphysema

Emphysema is one of the least understood and most destructive of all lung diseases. A lot of study needs to be done on this disease. Right now, it is considered to be a silent killer. It can utterly destroy people who are not even aware that they have it. It is detected only when it is in a progressive stage, when it has already done a lot of irreversible damage to the lungs.

Smoking is one of the culprits responsible for this disorder. If you observe any of its symptoms, quit smoking immediately and see a doctor. This is the only way to protect yourself from this ailment.

# Pregnancy Watch: What You Need To Know About Bronchitis

Pregnancy is an exciting moment for the would-be parents; a moment of great significance. It is the culmination of the love a man and woman have for each other. It also means that another individual is about to arrive into this world.

Pregnant women should take good care of themselves. Remember it is not just yourself your are taking care of; you are also taking care of your unborn baby. The immune system of an expecting mother is weakened, and therefore, she becomes susceptible to a myriad medical problems.

Usually, pregnant women suffer from colds and coughs. This is dangerous because colds and coughs can lead to more serious conditions such as bronchitis. Therefore, a pregnant woman must take special care to see that she does not catch a cold.

Bronchitis is a condition characterized by inflammation of the bronchioles. Its symptoms are similar to those of common cold. Keep away from conditions that might give you a cold if you are pregnant.

**Simple Way to Prevent Bronchitis**

To avoid contracting bronchitis, you need to avoid catching its symptoms. Put simply, it means that your simply cannot and should not catch a cold, and here is what you should do in order to avoid catching colds and coughs

Wash your hands as much and as often as possible. If you have to travel to a place where washrooms are not available, carry a hand sanitizer or alcohol.

Maintain cleanliness in and around your house. Things that you have to touch, especially, should be very clean. Invest in some germ-killing disinfectants and use them while cleaning your house.

**How To Win Your War Against Bronchitis**

Avoid people who have colds and coughs. In your present condition, you are highly susceptible to colds and coughs, and it is not advisable for you to interact with individuals suffering from a cold or cough.

# How Does Bronchitis Impact A Pregnant Woman?

Bronchitis can impact a pregnant woman is several ways.

A persistent cough is one of the symptoms of bronchitis. While it does your harm your baby, it can cause a lot of discomfort and annoyance to you.

Another symptom of bronchitis is a mild fever. According to medical studies, women who acquire a temperature higher than 38.9 degrees Celsius may give birth to a defective baby. So, if you get a high fever, it might impact your baby in adverse ways.

Symptoms such as cold, throat pain, and chest pain cause a great deal of annoyance to the pregnant woman; however, if checked at the right time, these symptoms won't cause any harm to your baby.

**Steps to be Taken if You Notice Symptoms of Bronchitis**

If you have observed the symptoms of bronchitis in yourself, you need to take necessary precautions to prevent the condition from becoming chronic. You also need to ensure that you do not suffer the discomforts that bronchitis can bring to a pregnant woman.

Drink plenty of non-caffeinated liquids because this eases mucus secretion. It is highly advisable for pregnant women suffering from bronchitis to drink plenty of water, fresh fruit juice, and soups.

Place a humidifier in your house; this will help you if you are suffering from cold.

Use saline drops to prevent stuffiness in your nose.

Take a warm shower daily. Studies have shown that a warm shower not only clears mucus but also prevents stuffiness in the nose.

Take plenty of rest. Relaxation is of utmost important.

**How To Win Your War Against Bronchitis**

Visit your obstetrician or gynecologist and talk to him or her about your condition.

**Medicines for Bronchitis**

It is not possible to avoid medicines even when you are pregnant. Medicines help you manage and control your condition better. Commonly, pregnant women with colds and allergies are treated with decongestants. Plenty of expectorants and cough suppressants are available to help pregnant women escape from the discomfort caused by coughing.

Before taking any of these medicines, however, remember to talk to your doctor. This way you can protect yourself and your unborn child.

# Battling With The Cough Symptoms In Chronic Bronchitis

A cough could be harmless; at the same time, it could be trying to convey a dangerous message. Only a physician will be able to unravel the mystery of a cough. For example, you will cough a lot if you have bronchitis; it is one of the symptoms of bronchitis. Knowledge about the various types and causes of a cough will help you determine the steps required to deal with cough.

## The Mechanism of a Cough

A cough is a simple body mechanism, characterized by a distinct sound, to get rid of any irritants that cause irritation to the air passages. When you cough, your thoracic cavity contracts abruptly, a movement that releases a lot of air from your lungs. The vagus nerve, which connects the lungs and the brain, has an important role to play in the mechanism of a cough.

## Why Do People Cough?

A cough is due to either physiological or psychological reasons. Psychological coughing is also called "habitual coughing." Those in the medical profession call it "streruphilia." An individual suffering from this condition enjoys sneezing or coughing, which is why he or she coughs or sneezes all the time.

On the contrary, a physiological cough is due completely to certain physiological conditions and can take place due to the following reasons:

- Bacterial, viral, or fungal infection leading to conditions such as common cold
- Allergy to irritating substances such as cigarette smoke, dust, pollen, or medicinal drugs
- Medical conditions such as coronary disorders, ear diseases, or sinuses in the lungs

# Types Of Cough

There are two types of cough--dry or non-productive cough and chesty or productive cough. A dry cough, which can cause a great deal of annoyance, is arid and stiff. In addition, it makes you feel tired and worn out. Usually, a bacteria or virus is responsible for a chesty cough. A chesty cough expels a lot of phlegm comprising mucus and germs from the respiratory system and, thereby, normalizes the breathing pattern.

## Effects of Cough in Chronic Bronchitis

Persistent, productive cough in chronic bronchitis can have the following effects:

- It causes strain in the anal region and, therefore, aggravates piles.
- Persistent coughing can sometimes lead to a headache.
- It causes additional strain in the stomach region, which can, in turn, lead to "scrotal sac" or hernia."
- It can raise the pressure in your chest and paves the way to a condition called "air emphysema."

## Controlling Cough in Chronic Bronchitis

According to medical studies, chronic bronchitis is chiefly due to smoking. Therefore, quit smoking immediately and for good if you are smoker. You will be surprised how fast your breathing pattern will return to normal once you stop smoking. Saying good-bye to cigarettes will not only reduce your cough but will also give you a pair of healthy lungs. In addition, keep away from a person who is smoking; the smoke can aggravate your cough. Medical studies have shown that passive smoking has worse effects on the lungs than active smoking.

Avoid irritants that can worsen your cough; some such irritants are chemical fumes, dust, and aerosol products. If you are inevitably exposed to irritants, wear a mask to avoid them.

If you have a persistent cough, visit your physician. He or she will help you determine the type of your cough. Your doctor is the best person to tell you the exact causes for your cough. In addition, a doctor is the most qualified person to teach you the best ways to prevent or treat that annoying cough. Therefore, the sooner you visit your physician, the better. Take no chances with your health!

# Pregnant Women With Bronchitis

A lot of changes take place in the body of woman when she is pregnant. She now needs plenty of oxygen and nutrients for the healthy growth and development of her unborn baby. A woman contracting bronchitis during pregnancy poses a gigantic medical challenge for physicians. While dealing with bronchitis during pregnancy, physicians have to take a number of factors into consideration. In this case, physicians have to:

- Take care of the health and well-being of pregnant women, whose bodies undergo a number of physiological and anatomical changes.
- Balance the requirements of the mother as well as the unborn infant.
- Deal with the pregnant woman's susceptibility to diseases.

## Dangers of Bronchitis During Pregnancy

Respiratory disorders, such as bronchitis during pregnancy, can cause intense suffering to a woman. In addition, the growing baby squeezes the diaphragm into the chest area, thereby reducing the amount of space available for the lungs and the size of the chest cavity. This makes it very difficult for the lungs to function effectively to supply oxygen to the mother and the unborn child. Serious damage can be caused to the child in the womb if sufficient oxygen is prevented from reaching it.

In addition, histologic evaluations of a pregnant woman's upper respiratory tract reveals conditions such as increased phagocytic activity, increased mucopolysaccharide content, hyperemia or rise in the amount of blood, and glandular hyperactivity or increased load of work on the glands.

## What is Bronchitis?

Bronchitis is a respiratory malady characterized by sputum production and a persistent cough. In bronchitis, the bronchial tree, comprising tubes that carry air into the lungs, is infected by bacteria, virus, or in rare cases, fungus. When these tubes get inflamed due to infection, they swell and secrete thick mucus. This accounts for the fact that people with bronchitis suffer from breathlessness.

## How To Win Your War Against Bronchitis

The two basic types of bronchitis are acute and chronic bronchitis. Acute bronchitis lasts for a short time and is caused by bacteria or viruses. Chronic bronchitis is caused by smoking or living in a highly polluted atmosphere.

The symptoms and signs of bronchitis are fatigue, abnormal sounds in the lungs or rales that a doctor can hear through a stethoscope, productive cough, pain in the chest, mild fever, wheezing, and difficulties in breathing

A number of tests are required before a patient can be diagnosed with the disease. Doctors use test results along with the visible signs and symptoms for proper diagnosis. The tests are to determine the nature of lung functioning, arterial blood gas, and sputum examinations; they also include chest x-ray and pulse oxymetry.

**Treatment of Bronchitis During Pregnancy**

Bronchitis during pregnancy is dealt in the same way as it is dealt in usual conditions. In particular situations, a few changes in treatment might be required. In addition, knowledge of the disease helps deal with bronchitis during pregnancy.

Antibiotics are prescribed if the cause of bronchitis is a bacteria. In case of virus-caused bronchitis, antibiotics are of no use. In usual conditions, doctors prescribe aspirin. However, aspirin is not prescribed in cases of bronchitis during pregnancy because it can cause bleeding and other complications.

No special treatment is required in case of acute bronchitis during pregnancy. The pregnant woman simply has to take a lot of rest, drink plenty of water and fruit juices, and use humidifiers in her house. It is important to keep away from cigarettes and cigarette smoke.

**Preventing Bronchitis During Pregnancy**

To repeat a worn-out saying, prevention is always better than cure. Pregnant women especially should be careful because they are more vulnerable to all sorts of disorders. Never smoke when you are pregnant; avoid smoke from other cigarettes. If your pregnancy comes during the

**How To Win Your War Against Bronchitis**

season of influenza, it is a good idea to take a flu vaccine. The vaccine might not be able to give you complete protection from bronchitis, but it will protect you from some types of virus that cause respiratory disorders.

# Medications That Can Battle Bronchitis

Basically, bronchitis is of two types--acute and chronic bronchitis. Although the names of the two are similar, there is a whale of a difference between them because they are caused by different agents. Therefore, there are different types of medicines for bronchitis.

## Acute Bronchitis

Acute bronchitis is common during the winter and does not last for a long time. A viral or a bacterial infection or both usually follows this condition. This disorder does not require any special treatment. It clears within a couple of weeks; however, the cough may persist for a longer time. There is a danger of acute bronchitis leading to pneumonia.

Elderly people, young children, and babies are the common victims of acute bronchitis. The immune systems of infants and young children are still in the growing phase, and this makes them susceptible to the disease while the immune systems of old people are weakened with age. Smokers and people who already have a lung or heart ailment stand the risk of contracting acute bronchitis. People living in polluted areas also commonly suffer from acute bronchitis.

## Medicines for Acute Bronchitis

First and foremost, the medicines for acute bronchitis aim to get rid of the symptoms of the disease.

People diagnosed with acute bronchitis need to drink plenty of water and fruit juices, stop smoking for good, take plenty of rest, relax as much as possible, and use humidifiers in their houses. The doctor prescribes medicines such as acetaminophen if the disease is accompanied by mild fever and pain. Sometimes, aspirin is also taken. However, pregnant women and children should not take aspirin because it is suspected to cause heavy bleeding in pregnant women and Reye's syndrome in children.

In case of dry cough, the patient can take an anti-cough medicine. But if it is cough accompanied by phlegm, it is advisable not to take any anti-cough medicine and to allow the body to cleanse itself. If such a cough is suppressed with an anti-cough medicine, the phlegm may accumulate in the lungs and host dangerous microbes. An expectorant is more advisable than an anti-cough medicine because it liquidities the thick mucus in the air passages and makes it easy for the patient to cough it out.

In case of bacterial infection, an antibiotic should be taken as prescribed by the doctor. A person who neglects to take antibiotics is in danger of suffering a relapse. In addition, the bacteria could produce a variant that is immune to medication. Antibiotic medicines include clarithromycin, azithromycin, trimethoprim or sulfamethazole, and so on. Children below the age of eight are given amoxillin instead of tetracyclin. Tetracyclin is suspected to cause discoloration of new teeth in young children.

## Chronic Bronchitis

Chronic bronchitis is characterized by inflammation of the respiratory tract. A common symptom is a persistent, productive cough that is accompanied by lots of phlegm. Unlike acute bronchitis, chronic bronchitis is a long-term disorder, and its symptoms are visible for three months to two years.

Inhalation of certain irritants may lie at the root of chronic bronchitis. Some examples of irritants are cigarette smoke or air pollution or a mixture of both. The disease progresses slowly, and the most common groups diagnosed with chronic bronchitis comprise the elderly and the middle-aged.

## Medicines for Chronic Bronchitis

Medicines for chronic bronchitis are different from those prescribed for acute bronchitis because it is a more complicated condition. Physicians carefully examine patients for other medical conditions before designing a treatment plan to control and manage the disease. Treatment also includes massive changes in lifestyle such as giving up smoking for good and moving to cleaner, non-polluted areas. Regular exercise also helps the patient deal with chronic bronchitis in a more effective manner.

The anti-inflammatory drugs that are commonly prescribed for chronic bronchitis are ipratropium, which reduces the production of mucus and coriticosteroids such as prednisone

**How To Win Your War Against Bronchitis**

that can be received either intravenously or orally. Bronchodilators such as metaproterenol and albuterol help loosen the bronchial muscles and this, in turn, increases the flow of air in the air passages. Bronchodilators can be either inhaled through a nebulizer, which is a medical device used to transport medication to the respiratory tract, or taken orally.

A person suffering from an advanced stage of chronic bronchitis might require supplemental oxygen. Hospitalization might be required if the patient has developed severe complications.

In addition to the usual medication, the treatment plan can also include herbal medicines. Herbs such as eucalyptus can be inhaled while a tea can be brewed from herbs such as mullein or verbascum thapsus, anise seed or Pimpinella anisum, and coltsfoot or Tussilago farfara.

A number of medicines for bronchitis are available. Don't take any of them on your own. Consult your physician, who is the best person to help you design a good treatment plan.

# Knowing The Difference Between Bronchitis And Pneumonia

It is very difficult to understand the differences between bronchitis and pneumonia. Both are diseases of the lower respiratory system and have an equally adverse effect on pulmonary air passages. Proper knowledge about the difference between pneumonia and bronchitis facilitates correct diagnosis, a factor that is of utmost importance in the effective management and treatment of respiratory disorders.

## What is Pneumonia?

Pneumonia is a severe infection of the lungs in which pus and other fluids fill the alveoli and prevent the free flow of air into the lungs. Due to this, the body does not get sufficient oxygen, and the cells are unable to function normally. Headache, excessive sweating, fatigue, and lack of appetite are some of the symptoms of pneumonia. The condition, if not treated with care, can cause death.

Several factors are responsible for pneumonia; however, the major causes of this condition are bacteria.

- Streptococcus pneumoniae causes community-acquired pneumonia in around 20-60 percent adults and 13-30 percent children.
- Group A or streptococcus pyogenes is also responsible for pneumonia.
- Staphylococcus aureus causes pneumonia in about 10-15 percent of hospitalized people. A fragile immune system and pre-existing viral influenza go hand in hand with this variety of pneumonia.
- Gram negative bacteria cause certain cases of community-acquired pneumonia. It also attacks people suffering from chronic lung disorders and children suffering from cystic fibrosis.

Certain viruses such as SARS (severe acute respiratory distress syndrome) virus, adenoviruses, herpes viruses, influenza viruses, RSV (respiratory syncytial virus), and HPV (human parainfluenza virus) also cause pneumonia.

# Types Of Pneumonia

There are different types of pneumonia.

**Atypical Pneumonia:** Bacteria are responsible for these types of pneumonia, including walking pneumonia. A person suffering from this variety could have a dry cough. It is a mild variety, and the patient need not be admitted to the hospital.

**Aspiration Pneumonia:** In this condition, bacteria are present in the oral cavity. If the bacteria remain in the oral cavity, they are harmless. However, if they penetrate the lungs, perhaps due to a weakening of the gag reflex, they could cause pneumonia.

**Opportunistic pneumonia:** As long as your immune system is in good condition, you don't have to worry about contracting this disease. However, people with weak immune systems should take special care not to get infected.

Regional and occupational pneumonia: For example, exposure to chemicals or cattle can cause this condition.

## What is Bronchitis?

Bronchitis is a disorder characterized by inflammation of the bronchi or air passages that transport air from the trachea to the lungs. Inflammation of the bronchi leads to the accumulation of mucus, which causes the blocking of the bronchial cells. The body then takes refuge in the cough mechanism to get rid of the accumulated mucus. Unfortunately, cough, while it gets rid of excess mucus, also makes the air passages more susceptible to infection. Moreover, if the infection continues, the tissues of the bronchi might get damaged.

## Types of bronchitis

Basically, there are two types of bronchitis--acute and chronic bronchitis.

**How To Win Your War Against Bronchitis**

**Acute bronchitis** is a short-term condition accompanied by a bad flu or a cold. It can keep you in a miserable condition for around two weeks. In certain cases, viral bronchitis can last for 8-12 weeks.

**Chronic bronchitis** is a long-term condition that can last anywhere from three weeks to two years. It always comes with a danger of relapse. In severe cases of chronic bronchitis, the bronchi get dilated, and this makes the patient more vulnerable to all types of infection. Due to its life-threatening nature, it should be taken seriously, and proper medical care should be taken to keep it in check.

**Causes and Treatment of Bronchitis**

Around ninety percent of the people contract acute bronchitis due to viral infection. Many cases are also caused due to bacterial infection. If you contract acute bronchitis many times, you might contract chronic bronchitis sooner or later. Infection need not always be the cause for acute bronchitis. If you live in a dirty, polluted area or if you a heavy smoker, you stand a greater risk of contracting chronic bronchitis.

If the condition is due to viral infection, polluted conditions, or heavy smoking, it is of no use taking antibiotics because they can do nothing to eliminate irritants or viruses. Antibiotics are useful only in case of bacterial infection.

It is possible to draw up any number of treatment plans for acute bronchitis. Follow your doctor's advice, avoid irritants, and adopt healthy patterns of lifestyle.

# Managing Bronchitis Symptoms And Knowing The Treatment

Bronchitis can easily be mistaken for a common cold. Dealing with bronchitis becomes easier once you learn to identify the various symptoms and signs of bronchitis.

There are two types of bronchitis--acute and chronic--and the symptoms of muscular aches, mild fever, chills, sore throat, insomnia, and breathlessness are common to both types of bronchitis; however, dyspnea is peculiar to chronic bronchitis.

## Basics of Bronchitis

Bronchitis is a condition in which viral or bacterial infection leads to inflammation of the respiratory tract. However, bacteria and virus are not always responsible for this condition. Continuous exposure to highly polluted atmospheres or a lifestyle trait such as heavy smoking renders the immune system so weak that the body becomes an ideal place for bacterial or viral infection.

Bronchitis usually begins with an infected sinus or a common cold. At first, the victims of bronchitis experience an irritating sensation in the posterior part of their throat, which is followed by a persistent cough accompanied by phlegm.

## Dealing with Cough

A common symptom of bronchitis is cough, which may be a dry cough or accompanied by phlegm. Cough accompanied by sputum generally indicates infection of the lower parts of the respiratory system.

In case of acute bronchitis, the patient may cough for a couple of weeks or more. Persistent cough causes a strain on the muscles of the abdomen and the thoracic cavity. If not treated properly and on time, persistent coughing might result in a damaged chest wall.

Since a cough might mean many things, a doctor will have to thoroughly examine the patient for any other medical condition that might be responsible for it. In case of severe, uncontrollable cough, the doctor might prescribe cough suppressants.

## Dealing with Other Symptoms

- Use a humidifier to deal with the uncomfortable feeling in the respiratory tract.
- Taking plenty of liquids helps cool the body temperature.
- In addition, liquid intake also helps liquefy the phlegm, and the body will find it easier to eliminate it via coughing. Expectorants such as quaifenesin also have the same effect.

## Medication for Bronchitis

In most cases, virus is responsible for this condition. Virus-caused bronchitis does not require any major treatment. It is easy to control and treat it at home. A few medicines, however, are taken to gain relief from the various symptoms.

## Antibiotics

Antibiotics are prescribed in cases of bacteria-caused bronchitis. However, an over dose of antibiotics will only make the bacteria more resistant to the medication.

Don't take antibiotics if the bronchitis is caused by virus or lifestyle patterns such as smoking or polluted environments because the antibiotics are of no use in such cases.

Antibiotics may also be used in case of patients suffering from long-term pulmonary disorders because their immune systems are so weak that they are susceptible to all sorts of bacterial infections.

## Pain Killers

Muscle pain is another symptom of this disorder. Pain killers such as aspirin and acetaminophen provide a lot of relief. However, an over dose of these drugs can cause gastric bleeding, and so, they should be taken on a full stomach.

**How To Win Your War Against Bronchitis**

Moreover, pregnant women and children are strictly not permitted to take these medicines. Aspirin is believed to cause Reye's syndrome in children. In pregnant women, it may result in severe bleeding.

**Other Medications**

Apart from the basic medication for bronchitis, doctors can prescribe medicines depending on the condition of individual patients.

Bronchodilators dilate the tissues of the respiratory tract to enable free flow of air. Consequently, they reduce wheezing. In extreme cases of chronic bronchitis, the patient might need additional oxygen to help him or her breathe.

In addition, patients are advised to take a flu vaccine along with a pneumococcal vaccine once in five or seven years. Mucolytic agents, alpha 1 antitrypsin therapy, and antitussive medications are also used in the treatment of bronchitis.

Herbal medicines that can be inhaled or taken in the form of a tea can also be used to alleviate the symptoms of bronchitis. However, it is crucial that you take herbal medication only after consulting your doctor.

# <u>Understanding The Foundation Of Chronic Bronchitis</u>

One of the manifestations of chronic bronchitis is a productive cough accompanied by phlegm, which obstructs the free flow of air in the bronchial tubes. Chronic bronchitis is a long-term disorder that can last as long as two years. It is the fourth largest killer in the United States of America, and around ten million people fall victim to this disorder every year. About 40,000 deaths due to chronic bronchitis have been recorded annually. It is considered to be the most common chronic obstructive pulmonary illnesses (CODP).

## Causes of Chronic Bronchitis

Certain lifestyle habits such as cigarette smoking are mainly responsible for chronic bronchitis. People who live in highly polluted atmospheres also fall prey to this disorder. The above-mentioned factors weaken the lungs and the body's immune system to such as extent that the person is easily infected by bacteria and viruses that attack the respiratory system.

Studies reveal that more than 90 percent of the people who contract chronic bronchitis comprise smokers. About 15 percent of the cigarette smokers are ultimately diagnosed with respiratory disorders characterized by obstruction of the airways. Biopsies of bronchial samples of people who have quit smoking thirteen years ago still reveal persistent marks of bronchial inflammation.

Tests conducted on patients suffering from chronic bronchitis reveal yet another disturbing factor--the presence of three varieties of bacteria: Moxarella catarrhalis, Haemophilus influenzae, and Streptococcus pneumoniae.

## Methods of Managing Chronic Bronchitis

Two methods of managing chronic bronchitis are in vogue at present--inhalation of ipratropium bromide and treatment through sympathomimetic agents. Theophyllinne is also an important therapy, but its uses are limited to a certain cases of the disorder. Patients who exhibit a remarkable improvement in airflow are not given any steriods. Antibiotics have a crucial part to play in the battle against acute infections. Supplemental oxygen is given to those patients who experience difficulties in breathing. Patients are also strongly advised to quit smoking for good, take plenty of nutritional supplements and fluids, and perform exercises to strengthen their respiratory muscles.

## Tests to Determine Chronic Bronchitis

A series of tests are necessary to determine a variety of factors. Needless to say, testing is also essential to make a correct diagnosis of the condition. The results of tests also confirm the extent to which the air passages are obstructed. Some of the tests include pulmonary function testing, blood tests, chest radiograph, electrocardiogram, biopsies, and sputum cultures.

The ratio between the measured forced expiratory volume (FEVI) and the forced vital capacity (FVC) defines the severity of chronic bronchitis. One of the signs of severe and long-term chronic bronchitis is progressive decline of FEVI rates. Factors such as age affect the elasticity of the lungs due to which the pulmonary testing of most adults over middle age show a 30ml decline in FEVI. In addition, the blocking of the bronchi due to an increase in the production of sputum does not always indicate chronic bronchitis. Pulmonary testing documents the reversible characteristics of air passage obstruction, and this helps physicians properly diagnose this disorder.

A sample of arterial blood is taken in order to do a blood test, which can determine conditions such as mild polychthemia.

Chest radiographs reveal conditions such as blebs, diaphragmatic flattening, peribronchial markings, hyperinflation, and bullae. However, the test results cannot be taken as final proof of the existence of chronic bronchitis.

Electrocardiograms pinpoint disturbances, such as arterial fibrillation or flutter and atrial tachycardia having "P" pulmonale, in the supraventricular rhythm.

Airway biopsies can reveal submucosal and mucosal inflammation, hyperplasia of goblet cells, and abnormal smoothness of the muscles on the small noncartilaginous air passage.

Sputum culture is done in case of patients who have not been hospitalized but display acute exacerbations of chronic bronchitis. It is one of the methods used to determine the requirement for antibiotic therapy. Protected-tip sputum cultures are done in case of patients who are in hospitals especially if atypical organisms are suspected to cause the exacerbation.

Mortality rate after the diagnosis of chronic bronchitis is fifty percent. The terminal event of chronic bronchitis is respiratory failure. Respiratory failure is due to bacterial infections characterized by purulent sputum, fever, and poor ventilation symptoms. The other factors responsible for respiratory failure are seasonal changes, infections of the upper respiratory system, medications, and prolonged exposure to polluting and irritating agents.

An understanding of the factors responsible for inflammation in chronic bronchitis makes it easier to manage, control, and treat this disorder.

# Tell-Tale Signs Of Chronic Bronchitis

The term "bronchitis" is derived from two Greek words "bronchos" and "itis," which mean "windpipe" and "inflammation," respectively. True to its name, bronchitis is a respiratory disorder characterized by inflammation of the windpipe and the large and small bronchi due to bacterial or viral infection or factors such as environmental pollution or cigarette smoking.

Chronic bronchitis is the more lethal of the two types of bronchitis, that is, acute and chronic bronchitis. While acute bronchitis lasts for a short time and is chiefly caused by bacterial or viral infection, chronic bronchitis lasts much longer. It is also considered to be one of the chronic obstructive pulmonary disease (COPD), a group of respiratory diseases commonly characterized by abnormal breathing patterns.

**Recognizing Chronic Bronchitis**

If the patient coughs and expels sputum for about three months in a year for two consecutive years, the patient might be suffering from chronic bronchitis. Chronic bronchitis is also characterized by excessive production of mucus, cough, and dysnea, or difficulties in breathing while exerting oneself physically.

Chronic bronchitis is accompanied by abnormal signs in the lungs, edema of the feet, coronary failure, and a bluish tinge on the skin and around the lips. The symptoms disappear with the passage of time and are usually followed by the development of abnormal breathing patterns.

Dyspnea, characterized by labored breathing, interferes a lot with the sufferers' daily routine. It turns out that breathing takes up all of a person's energy. Subsequently, the patients lose a lot of weight because even the normal process of eating involves a major expenditure of energy.

Due to dyspnea, even the slightest exertion will be exhausting for the person. As chronic bronchitis progresses, patients experience difficulties in breathing even when they are taking rest. At this stage, patients become more susceptible to infections of all types and to respiratory insufficiencies, which pave the way for the terminal event of chronic bronchitis, acute respiratory failure.

These symptoms might be similar to the symptoms of other respiratory disorders, which is why patients must never try to diagnose the condition on their own. Consulting a doctor is of utmost importance. It is possible to mistake chronic bronchitis for other respiratory disorders such as asthma, sinusitis, tuberculosis, pulmonary emphysema, and so on.

## Various Medical Tests to Diagnose Chronic Bronchitis

Physicians conduct a number of tests to facilitate correct diagnose of a respiratory condition. Some of the tests and examinations are:

Pulmonary function tests are done to calculate the capacity of the lungs to exchange oxygen for carbon-di-oxide. In order to conduct pulmonary function tests, doctors use peak flow monitoring (PFM) and spirometry. Spirometry is a medical tool used to determine and understand the working of the lungs while PFM is used to determine the maximum speed with which a person can exhale or inhale. PFM also assesses the ways in which the malady can be controlled.

Pulse oxImetry Is a small apparatus that measures the oxygen content in the blood.

Chest x-rays are a common diagnostic tool to view pictures of the internal conditions of organs, tissues, and bones.

Arterial Blood Gas (ABG) is the name of a blood test to ascertain the capacity of the lungs to supply oxygen to the body and to eliminate carbon-di-oxide from it. In addition, it helps measure the acid content of the blood.

Computed Tomography or CT Scan is a medical technique that combines x-ray and computer technology to obtain a comprehensive image of different parts of the human body.

Chronic bronchitis usually lasts throughout life, and treatment is taken only to alleviate its distressing symptoms. In spite of this, the patient can live a comfortable, productive life by properly managing the symptoms of this disease. The disorder, though incurable, is controllable.

# Bronchitis: The Drugs That Can Help Treat Bronchitis

Modern society suffers mostly from various kinds of respiratory disorders, some contagious and some noncontagious. The markets are flooded with a variety of drugs to treat bronchitis and other disorders. All of us need to have adequate knowledge about how to maintain good health. We need to know the best drugs to treat bronchitis, in case we are stricken with it.

Bronchitis, a respiratory disorder that can affect anybody at anytime, is one among the most widespread ailments. However, people residing in polluted areas, cigarette smokers, infants, young children, old people, and people already suffering from lung disorders are more susceptible to bronchitis.

**Treatment of Acute Bronchitis**

Acute bronchitis is the milder of the two types of bronchitis. There is no need to take any drugs to treat bronchitis of this type, which is a short-term disorder. Acute bronchitis lasts only for a couple of weeks or lesser if treated with care. The duration of the illness also depends on the type of microbe causing it.

However, some patients take expectorants to facilitate easier breathing. Anti-inflammatory drugs will help you obtain relief from the various symptoms of bronchitis. In certain cases, bronchitis can lead to very painful sinusitis. Decongestants will help you alleviate this symptom. You might also require pain killers to ease the muscle pain that always comes with bronchitis.

There is no need to take any drugs to treat bronchitis that is caused by viruses. You simply need a lot of rest, water and fruit juices in abundance, and a humidifier. In addition, you have to avoid dust and polluted environments. The only drugs required in this conditions are those that alleviate the symptoms of bronchitis--anti-inflammatory drugs, pain killers, expectorants, and nasal decongestants.

You have to take antibiotics or antibacterial drugs to treat bronchitis that is caused by bacteria; the drugs destroy the bacteria that are infecting your bronchi. In rare cases, the bronchitis might be caused by a fungus, and you will have to take antifungal drugs in addition to the other medicines that tackle the symptoms of bronchitis.

## How To Win Your War Against Bronchitis

Along with the medication and the rest of the treatment plan, it is essential that you stop smoking. The earlier you quit smoking, the sooner you can undo the damage done to your lungs.

## Treatment of Chronic Bronchitis

On the other hand, chronic bronchitis, a long-term disorder, requires long-term care. If you are suffering from chronic bronchitis, you need to take a variety of drugs to obtain relief from the symptoms of the disorders along with drugs that might help cure the condition.

Some of the medicines typically taken by patients suffering from chronic bronchitis are bronchodilators to dilate the bronchi and to enable easier breathing, antibiotics to destroy any bacteria that might be infecting your respiratory tract, and steroids. In certain cases, people suffering from chronic bronchitis require supplemental oxygen to help them deal with the low levels of oxygen in their body.

Chances for complete recovery from chronic bronchitis are slim. You need to identify the disease in its earliest stages and arrest its further progress immediately. You can do so by making major lifestyle changes such as moving to a cleaner area, quitting smoking, and giving up alcohol altogether.

Before taking any sort of drug to treat bronchitis, consult your doctor. Your doctor will determine, on the basis of your medical history, whether or not a particular drug will be beneficial for you. Doctors are the most qualified to determine the best combination of drugs to treat bronchitis. They also give you the correct instruction about the usage of these drugs.

# Herbal Remedy For Bronchitis: A Natural Way To Treat Bronchitis

Generally, people have a good reason to develop a variety of medicines for a variety of medical disorders Everyone wants a healthy body and to live happy, normal, and productive lives. At the same time, it is impossible to be always healthy. With so many bacteria and virus around, it is quite normal to get infected by a bacteria or virus.

Bronchitis is known to be one among the world's most common respiratory disorders. It is characterized by inflammation of the bronchial tubes, and can disrupt its victims' day-to-day lives. Fortunately, there are many herbal cures for bronchitis.

There are two types of bronchitis--acute and chronic. Virus, bacteria, or fungus are responsible for acute bronchitis. The signs of acute bronchitis include mild chest pain, low grade fever, sinusitis, pressure around the areas of the eyes, persistent productive cough, wheezing, fatigue, and discomfort in the chest.

Acute bronchitis is easy to manage, control, and treat. When properly treated, it lasts for not more than a couple of weeks and is usually followed by flu or common cold. As soon as you recognize these symptoms in yourself or a loved one, visit your doctor. Physicians can determine whether your condition is caused by a bacteria, virus, or fungus. After diagnosing the condition accurately, a doctor is in a position to prepare the perfect treatment plan for you.

Virus-caused acute bronchitis doesn't require any special medication to bring about a cure. You could consider taking a few drugs, such as anti-inflammatory drugs, decongestants, expectorants, and pain killers, in order to obtain relief from bronchitis symptoms. The addition of a few herbal cures for bronchitis forms an ideal treatment plan.

Never take any drugs without first consulting your doctor. This is because you might have an allergy to a particular type of drug. Moreover, some drugs, such as aspirin, are dangerous for pregnant women and children, especially when taken in combination with other types of drugs.

## How To Win Your War Against Bronchitis

Research has shown that many herbal cures for bronchitis that are highly effective in giving relief from the distressing symptoms of bronchitis. Consider the following herbal cures if you are suffering from bronchitis:

Eucalyptus oil can help alleviate cough. It liquefies the phlegm and makes it easy for the body to expel it from the lungs. A number of physicians from different parts of the world advise bronchitis patients to use eucalyptus.

Garlic is yet another herbal remedy that can prevent, or at least lessen the chances of contracting bronchitis. Eat plenty of garlic; it contains chemicals that are anti-virus and anti-bacterial. To put it differently, garlic is an excellent natural antibacterial and antiviral herb.

Recently, studies have shown that the stinging variety of nettle has the properties to cure bronchitis and other forms of respiratory disorders. Drink the juice of its roots and leaves along with sugar or honey.

Take plenty of herbal sources of vitamin C.
Herbs that contain magnesium can also help bronchitis patients.
Drink the juice of regano leaves.

The best method to prevent bronchitis is to make major lifestyle changes such as giving up cigarettes and alcohol. If you live in a polluted region, move to a cleaner zone. Regular exercises are essential to maintain the health of your respiratory system.

Many times, acute bronchitis is mistaken to be common cold. A doctor is the only person who can tell the difference. So, if you suspect that you have contracted bronchitis, visit the doctor and get your condition properly diagnosed so that an effective treatment plan can be prepared. Neglect to do this might lead to complications such as chronic bronchitis, which will leave you disabled for life.

# <u>How To Treat Bronchitis: Ten Simple Steps Plus Useful Advice Works</u>

Bronchitis is a disorder of the respiratory system characterized by inflammation of the windpipe and the bronchi. Viral or bacterial infection is responsible for acute bronchitis. On the other hand, chronic bronchitis is caused when the lungs are continuously irritated by cigarette smoke or exposure to polluted or hazardous conditions.

Do not despair if your doctors tell you that you have contracted bronchitis. The following ten steps will tell you how to successfully treat bronchitis:

1.	Get away from irritants, pollutants, and toxins that are causing havoc to your lungs. Quit smoking for good and avoid being a passive smoker too. In case you live in a polluted area, either move to a cleaner place or keep within the confines of your home. Protect yourself form hazardous substances and other irritants by wearing a face mask.

2.	Keep a humidifier or a vaporizer inside your house to increase the humidity of your immediate environment. This will help you breathe more easily.

3.	Keep a hot water bottle or a hot, moist cloth against your chest or back. This serves to reduce inflammation and is highly effective if done at bed time.

4.	If you are planning a visit to cooler areas, remember to cover your nose and mouth with a warm handkerchief. This precaution has to be taken because cold conditions aggravate bronchitis.

5.	Do not take cough suppressants. Coughing is the body's way of throwing out unwanted secretions. You may, however, take a suppressant at night, to facilitate a good night's sleep.

6.	Take your medicines as prescribed by your doctor. If your condition is due to bacterial infection, you will have to take antibiotics. Do not miss any dose. Complete the entire course of medication even if you feel that you are getting better.

## How To Win Your War Against Bronchitis

7.      Use aerosols and inhalers as prescribed by your doctor. Don't increase the dose because it might cause harmful side effects.

8.      You may have to take dietary supplements such as colloidal silver, zinc, vitamins C and A, coenzyme Q10, goldenseal, and echinacea. However, before taking anything, consult your doctor.

9.      Plan a nutritious, well-balanced diet. Drink plenty of liquids such as soups, herbal tea, fruit juices, and water.

10.     Do not take foods that might encourage mucus production. A list of such foods includes dairy products, white flour, processed foods, sugar, and foods that cause allergy.

In addition to the above ten steps, people suffering from bronchitis usually use the following methods to treat bronchitis:

Eat cucumber mixed with vinegar. It effectively cleans out the excess mucus. In addition, it also helps kill the bacteria that are infecting the lungs.

Take a charcoal slush comprising a mixture of 4-6 teaspoons of charcoal powder mixed with water. It does not taste foul and you can easily drink it. Take a dose of this slush every 4-6 hours when you are awake. The charcoal absorbs bacteria and other harmful germs and will be harmlessly eliminated by the body in the bathroom.

Frankincense, oregano, and thyme oils help relieve breathlessness. Take two drops of frankincense oil mixed with Ciaga's organic juice thrice a day for three days. At the end of the third day, take oregano and thyme oils in a similar manner. You can even use pleurisy root as an alternative.

Boil water in a vessel full of aromatic herbs. Wrap your head with a towel. Cover the vessel with part of the towel and breathe in the aromatic fumes. Do this many times a day at intervals. This practice will help liquefy the phlegm.

**How To Win Your War Against Bronchitis**

Pound the patient's back gently while he or she is lying on his or her belly with the body's upper portion in a hanging position. This breaks down or dislocates the phlegm. This procedure is neither comfortable nor safe. However, if done correctly, it is an excellent way of getting rid of the mucus that blocks the air passages.

Consult a doctor if the symptoms last more than a week. If the mucus turns yellow, green, or rust-colored, it is a sign of danger and requires the attention of a physician. Before making any changes to your diet or taking any nutritional supplements, consult your doctor or health care provider. The information provided in the article is to be used along with the usual medication because it, in no way, serves as an efficient substitute for a doctor's treatment or advise.

# Is Bronchitis Contagious: Clearing Your Mind From Doubts

To know whether bronchitis is contagious or not, you need to know something about the types, causes, and symptoms of the disorder.

## What is Chronic Bronchitis?

In chronic bronchitis, there is inflammation of the mucosal membranes of the bronchial tubes due to infection, a condition that leads to an excess in the production of mucus. This extra mucus disrupts normal breathing processes by blocking the air passages and preventing the entry of sufficient quantity of air into the lungs.

## Symptoms of Chronic Bronchitis

The symptoms of chronic bronchitis include difficulty in breathing, breathlessness, wheezing, pain in the chest, productive cough, and discomfort. The typical chronic bronchitis cough, intense and persistent, is also known as "smoker's cough." These symptoms are persistent and intensify as the disease progresses. During the initial stages of bronchitis, patients notice its symptoms either in the evening or in the morning.

Chronic bronchitis is usually accompanied by pulmonary problems such as pneumonia and emphysema. With the passage of time, chronic bronchitis patients suffer from poor oxygenation and hypoventilation. Lack of oxygen results in cyanosis, a condition characterized by a bluish tinge on the skin that suggests the presence of pneumonia or emphysema.

## Difficulties of Treating Chronic Bronchitis

Medical science has still not found appropriate medicines to cure this condition. It focuses on relieving the symptoms of this condition in order to prevent it from proceeding to more complicated stages. The disease can last for three months a year for two consecutive years, and there can always be a relapse.

People suffering from chronic bronchitis are more susceptible to all sorts of infection and do not respond easily to medication. The condition does not respond to antibiotics as well as acute bronchitis does. This is because the excess mucus produced by the bronchial tubes is an excellent ground for the rapid multiplication of bacteria and other infection-causing organisms.

**Causes of Bronchitis**

Smoking is not the only major cause of chronic bronchitis although the ailment is commonly seen among regular smokers. Smoking in itself does not cause the disease; but it facilitates the multiplication of bacteria and thereby slows the healing process in the respiratory tissues. Continuous exposure to pollutants such as hazardous chemicals, smoke, or dust is responsible for chronic bronchitis.

When acute bronchitis is neglected or wrongly treated, it often progresses to chronic bronchitis or some other pulmonary disorder. On the other hand, infection of the lungs is responsible for acute bronchitis. About ten percent of acute bronchitis is bacterial while ninety percent is viral. When a person is continuously affected by acute bronchitis, his or her bronchial tubes are weakened, and this paves the way for chronic bronchitis.

Factors such as industrial pollution are also responsible for chronic bronchitis. Most patients of chronic bronchitis are coal miners, metal molders, and grain handler. Many of them work in the midst of dust. Atmospheres high in sulfur dioxide can also aggravate the symptoms of chronic bronchitis.

**How Contagious is Bronchitis?**

Certain types of bronchitis such as asthmatic bronchitis are not contagious because virus or bacteria have no role to play here. This condition is contagious only when bacteria or virus are transferred from person to person by direct or indirect contact. When an infected person coughs or sneezes, fluid from his or her nose or mouth can spread to others around him or her.

Bronchitis can also spread when common vessels and drinking glasses are shared or when handkerchiefs or tissues used by an infected person are touched.

Since viruses complete their life cycle in a few days, bronchitis that follows a viral cold is not contagious. However, the condition is contagious if the patient still displays symptoms of cold.

**How To Win Your War Against Bronchitis**

If the person has been suffering from the condition for more than ten days, there is no danger of the condition being contagious; this is the aftermath of bronchitis.

Healthy people only need to take care to prevent getting infected. Beware of infectious particles when a person suffering from bronchitis coughs; you could then catch the infection.

# Prevention Of Acute Bronchitis – 11 Easy Tips

Health is Wealth – this is what the wise men suggest and stands true in all regards.

Having loads of wealth and no health to enjoy and make fun in life makes no sense. Similarly to earn wealth you need proper health. Hence keeping healthy is the basic key to success.

In the lifestyle that we lead today we are surrounded with so much pollution and unwanted, unhygienic factors that it is a must to be cautious enough keep the ailments away form yourself. In short your health entirely lies in your own hands.

One of the most common ailments these days is the respiratory ailment. Asthma being the most known respiratory disease there are several others alongside that you must be aware of. One such ailment is bronchitis.

Bronchitis is a sort of a respiratory illness affecting the bronchial tree of our body. That is, in this ailment bronchi of our lungs becomes inflamed. It is a common disease among tobacco smokers & people ho are living in the areas where there are high levels of air pollution. In case you one among those affected with bronchitis, here are some points you must understand about this disease.

1. Bronchitis is of two kinds depending on the time it lasts for in the body - Acute bronchitis lasts for only 10-12 days. On the other hand, chronic bronchitis might also take 3 months to 2 years.

2. It is easier to prevent acute bronchitis because it is mainly caused due to some viral & bacterial infections.

3. Also there are some cases where this ailment comes from some fungus. The individual suffering with acute bronchitis experiences persistent cough along with mucus, shortness of breathe, feeling of fatigue, mild fever, mild chest pains, feeling of coldness, vibration inside chest while breathing, etc.

4. When acute bronchitis is caused due to virus, it is usually the same virus as that of common cold. In case of such viral infections, the doctors suggest that there is no need of any special medications. The only means of getting well is talking lots of rest and drinking loads of non caffeinated & non alcoholic beverages.

5. In case one is affected with acute bronchitis caused due to the bacterial infection, the usual antibiotic medications can treat him/her well. In such remember two things – one contact the doctor and take the anti-biotic that the expert suggests rather than taking just any medicine without prescription and two, increasing the humidity in the patients' house would really help. You can do this by placing wet towels all across the house or placing room humidifiers.

6. Generally, acute bronchitis lasts about 10-12 days only. Yet, it is closely followed and/or associated with flu and cold. So, many a times during the healing process coughing does not end and bronchi in the lungs keeps irritating. In case the coughing lasts longer than a month, the experts advise you to consult the physician immediately, before the conditions get worst. This is because, cough occurs for several other reasons as well.

As the wise men say, prevention is better than cure, here are some easy tips to prevent the bronchial diseases:

1. Wash your hands more often that too every time very thoroughly.

2. The smokers must understand that smoking can increase this ailment to vast extent, so they must quit smoking immediately in order to prevent this disorder.

3. Our environment now a days is filled with extremely polluted air. So you must invest in some air conditioners, curtains and filters for your home to purify the air as much as possible.

4. Bronchitis, the respiratory illness can affect you any time, any where, and at times we do not even come to know about the ailment. So you must understand the signs & symptoms of this disease in order to know when ever you become a victim to it. In case

**How To Win Your War Against Bronchitis**

of any information you need, do not delay getting to your doctor and seeking some valuable knowledge.


5.  Remember, bronchitis is preventable provided you decide to live a healthy & hygienic lifestyle.

# Antibiotics For Bronchitis - 6 Common Prescriptions

An antibiotic is a type of medication that is prescribed to a patient to destroy and/or put off the growth of bacteria. Depending on the infection you are afflicted with, the anti-biotic is given to the patient.

Bronchitis is a respiratory disease in which the air passageway between our nose & lungs inflames. It is of two type – short term or acute, long term or chronic. Chronic bronchitis is a worst condition for any individual to be in.

The antibiotics when prescribed in the cases of bronchitis do not exactly treat bronchitis. They decrease the infections that aggravate the symptoms of the ailment. The medical experts explain that some antibiotics have been great help in decreasing the cough just after one or two weeks of decreasing the infection in the patient.

Some antibiotics quite commonly used to cure the acute & chronic bronchitis are as follows:

## 1. Ampicillin

This is used to treat the infections developed with acute bronchitis. In case you are prescribed this medicine, you must take a glass full of water with in 30 minutes or 2 hours, after having the meals.

Amcipillin's usual side effects include skin irritation, diarrhea, soreness of the tongue and/or mouth, vomiting, etc.

This medicine is most oft given to the adults.

## 2. Trimethoprim

This antibiotic is primarily used to cure the respiratory tract's infections. Other uses of trimethoprim include treatment of urine & ear infections.

Some of the commonly known side effects of this anti-biotic are stomach pain, diarrhea, swollen tongue, and sometimes it can lead to the failure of having proper diet due to difficulty in eating properly.

Some types of pills included under this header are – Septra, Bactrim, etc.

## 3. Azithromycin

This one is most oft used to treat the patients suffering with bacterial infections arising bronchitis & pneumonia.

It is taken in the form of a tablet and also in the form of oral suspension.

The side effects of Azithromycin include:
i. Irritated stomach
ii. Loose bowel movement
iii. Vomiting
iv. Pain in the patients' stomach & abdomen
v. Skin irritations like rashes that are usually minor

The usual brands manufacturing this antibiotic are Zitromax, Aztrin, and Zmax.

## 4. Amoxicillin

This drug is quite commonly prescribed one for many ailments.  Amoxicillin is aailbale in the form of capsules, tablets (that are chewable for children), liquid suspension, pediatric drops, etc.

Its side effects include irritated stomach, diarrhea, vomiting, etc. In extreme cases this medication leads to some very severe side effects like atypical bleeding, seizures, & too much fatigue.

The brands that manufacture this type of antibiotic are Trimox, Amoxil, Sumox, etc.

This one is usually prescribed for the young children inflicted with bronchitis.

## 5. Telithromycin

While chronic bronchitis is quite a serious ailment and needs a very vital treatment, telithromycin is commonly used to treat it now a days.

This anti-biotic primarily ministers over the mild and moderate infections occurring in the course of respiratory system functions.

The brand name linked with this anti-biotic is Ketek.

This medication can be taken in the form of a tablet or the oral suspension.

The commonly known side effects of this medication are lightheadedness, headache, irritated stomach, loose bowel movement, blunt taste, unclear vision, etc.

## Safety Precautions While Taking Antibiotics

In case you are diagnosed to have bronchitis and now it has become a must for you to have anti-biotics, there are many precautions that you must take in order to minimize the side effects. Bronchitis and the other infections can be relieved very effectively with the specific & prescribed antibiotics, given that you take them in the prescribed manner. The ways to deal with the common side effects are as follows:

1. Be precise while informing your physician regarding the severity of the extent of bronchitis. This would enable them to decide as to you must take the antibiotic or not and if yes which type you must take.

2. Make sure to mention clearly about the allergies you have with any all sort of elements, mainly food & medicines.

3. Be sure to complete the dosage prescribed by the doctor and not leave it in the midst else the infection would continue to persists in the body.

**How To Win Your War Against Bronchitis**

4. In case you have missed a dose, make sure to take it and get to the normal cycle, soon enough.

5. In case the patient is pregnant, you must consult the OB-GYNE to check if the medicines are suited to your condition.

6. When the side effects rise too much, consult you physician as he may change or stop the medication.

7. The medications have their own advantages & disadvantages. If the dosage is taken well enough with the help of the caregiver or some family member it would show up all positives and minimum negatives.

# Asthmatic Bronchitis - 25 Points To Remember

Bronchitis is quite a known chronic disease. Basically bronchitis implies irritation & inflammation in the bronchial tubes along with the neighboring organs & tissues that our body uses for breathing.

The bronchial tubes in the human body filter the air passing through the respiratory tract while it sets out for the lungs. The bronchial tubes are covered with some minute hair-like projections that prevent the dirt and/or irritants (like dust and/or pollen) from entering the essential parts of our respiratory tract. The hair-like projections are termed as cilia.

The long term contact with viruses, chemicals, and/or even dust particles facilitates the irritants to shatter the natural defenses of our respiratory system, eventually causing infection & inflammation.

## Asthmatic Bronchitis

1. Also known as COPD, the asthmatic bronchitis is a pulmonary disease.

2. COPD stands for Chronic Obstructive Pulmonary Disease.

3. It typically affects the individuals who are suffering with chronic bronchitis.

4. It is not easy to differentiate asthmatic bronchitis from the other lung diseases. This is due to the symptoms that are quite similar in both the cases.

5. The symptoms of asthmatic bronchitis resemble those of several other respiratory tract diseases such as bronchitis, sinusitis, common asthma, and emphysema.

6. Asthma is the persistent inflammatory disease in the respiratory tract of the human body where our airway passages become extra sensitive, produce excessive mucus, and the mucus edema.

7.  The key difference between the other obstructive lung diseases and asthmatic bronchitis is that the latter is often reversible, both, with or without the treatment.

8.  Persons afflicted with asthma might experience certain symptom free episodes while interchanging acute asthmatic attacks last for a few minutes or a few days.

9.  Factors setting off the asthmatic attacks are quite similar to the asthmatic bronchitis (like dust, smoking, etc.).

10.  Common asthma is mainly triggered through the allergens. The common allergens imply ones arising due to season (that is weed pollens and grass tree), and the persistent ones (like roaches, animal dander, dust, etc). Almost all asthmatic individuals are extremely sensitive to these triggers.

11.  The key causes of bronchitis are the bacterial infections. While asthmatic bronchitis is activated through tiny specks breaking through the safety walls created by cilia, a part of the bronchial tubes.

12.  Just like other COPDs, the asthmatic bronchitis involves congestion of our respiratory tract. The bronchial tubes actually produce mucus under all normal circumstances. This mucus then covers our lungs, trachea, and other important organs of the respiratory system. When the irritants are existent in our respiratory system, there is an overproduction of this mucus that consequently obstructs our airways. A continuous mucoid obstruction in the respiratory tract is the most common factor among the asthmatic bronchitis patients.

13.  These factors contribute towards the development of the asthmatic bronchitis, hyperactivity of bronchus and/or immunologic aberrations, the relentless childhood infections, etc.

14.  The persons suffering with asthma and/or the other grave sorts of chronic bronchitis become quite vulnerable towards asthmatic bronchitis.

15.  Ones who are afflicted with the chronic bronchitis, ultimately contract to asthmatic bronchitis owing to the long term exposure towards pollutants and/or environmental toxins & mainly cigarette smoking.

16.   While the medical experts continue to research what exactly causes this disease by far the established fact is that the environmental factors lead to this ailment.

17.   The general symptoms leading to asthmatic bronchitis include dyspnea (that is difficulty in breathing & shortness of breath), chest discomforts, cough, wheezing lasting for several weeks, general malaise or fatigue, weight loss, pain, usual feeling of soreness, high risk to catch infections, etc.

18.   While the above mentioned factors are also seen in the common asthmatic patients, the persons suffering with asthmatic bronchitis also show rather profound symptoms. These are those symptoms that show higher frequencies as compared to a common asthma.

19.   One important symptom is the person faces problems reaching the high or low music notes while singing.

20.   The medical treatment given for asthmatic bronchitis is almost similar to that given in the case of chronic bronchitis. The medications in both the cases involve steroids, anti-biotics and bronchodilators.

21.   Though these medications only help in alleviating the symptoms & comforting the patient as much as possible. They do not exactly cure the disease.

22.   Often the patients of asthmatic bronchitis have to take long term treatments in order to improve their health. The doctors counsel tem on how to keep away from irritants like pollen, dust, chemicals, alcohol fumes, smoke, etc.

23.   Such patients must also avoid the bacterial infections by not going in to the crowds. In case this becomes unavoidable, the patients must wear masks covering their mouth & nose.

24.   Such patients are always required to take influenza vaccines.

25.   They must educate themselves about he precautionary measures so as to avoid all further bacterial or viral infections.

# Bronchitis Among Children - 20 Points To Remember

Bronchitis is a respiratory ailment that can happen at all ages. It scares all the parents as they do not want their children to be afflicted with the ailment. A key identification of this ailment is inflammation of a person's bronchi that is a part of our lungs.

First of all, the parents and/or caregivers can calm down as the medical findings have proved that bronchitis among children is not a chronic ailment.

Though among children bronchitis is certainly not a chronic ailment, the parents and/or caregivers must essentially acquire the knowledge on the disease. This way they would be able to help their child better while the child suffers a bronchitis attack.

In the disease of bronchitis, the air passages amidst the child's lungs & nose swell up owing to the viral infection. This affects the child's bronchi. Bronchi refer to the tubes where in the air passes through in to & out of the child's lungs. Many a times, the tracheas & windpipe are also affected by this inflammation.

**Bronchitis is of two types - acute & chronic**

Acute bronchitis or the short term bronchitis is perhaps the most common among bronchial ailments. Chronic bronchitis usually appears among the adults. The ones who smoke heavily and/or are prone to inhaling the chemical substances have quite many chances to catch chronic bronchitis.

**Acute Bronchitis**

1.  This type of bronchitis is the most common one for the winter season, especially among children.

2.  The viruses attack the child's lining of bronchial tree that leads to infection. The swelling heightens as the child's body combats with the attack of the viruses.

3.  As the swelling increases, more & more mucus is produced in the body.

4.  The child is most likely to develop acute bronchitis in case the causative virus of the ailment is inhaled in the air that they breathe or it can get passed over from a person coughing.

5.  Therefore, the ailment of acute bronchitis is most oft acquired by the air the child breathes.

6.  The symptoms & signs of acute bronchitis among children are:

    i. Runny nose
    ii. Followed by cough
    iii. Slight fever
    iv. Experiencing pain in the back & muscle area
    v. Sore throat
    vi. Getting chills
    vii. Malaise

7.  In the early stage of acute bronchitis, the child suffers with dry & unproductive cough. This later on develops in to copious cough all filled with mucus. In some cases, the child vomits or gags as he/she coughs.

8.  In case you notice the symptoms given above in the children, the experts say, it is high time that you should take the child to the physician. Initially the doctor does a physical examination and refers to the child's medical history to conclude whether he is suffering with the said ailment or not.

9.  To verify the ailment developing in the child, the following tests are referred to by the medical practitioners:

    i. Blood tests
    ii. X-ray of the chest
    iii. Lung Tests
    iv. Pulse Oximetry

v.Sputum cultures

10. To cure the acute bronchitis among children the key word is taking rest. You must ensure that the child takes a good & well balanced meal. Also, drinking loads of non-caffeinated fluids is very helpful. Another key tip to cure this ailment is maintaining the in the surroundings of the child.  You can do this by placing room humidifiers or keeping wet towels in several places in the house.

11. Some times the medical practitioners recommend some asthma related medications for the child. These medications help the child release the mucus jammed inside the child's bronchi tubes. Usually with these medications an inhaler is also prescribed.

12. To relieve the child's fever and the feeling of discomfort, analgesics are also a part of the prescription.

13. The parents and/or caregivers must note that hey should not give aspirin to the child who is suffering with bronchitis. This can lead to devastating results and other ailments like Reye's syndrome.

14. Along side, antihistamines must also be prevented as these can worsen the cough of the child.

15. In order to avoid recurring acute bronchitis for the child, you must ensure that the child washes his hands well regularly.

16. Also make sure that the child keeps away from all sorts of smokes like that coming from the belches or cigarettes.

## Chronic Bronchitis

1.  When the bronchial symptoms persistently afflict the individual for three months or more, it is termed as chronic bronchitis.

2.  This usually initiates with a continuous irritation in the bronchial tubes.

**How To Win Your War Against Bronchitis**

3.  Among children, acute bronchitis is rather common as compared to the chronic type of the ailment. The studies prove that chronic bronchitis hits the children usually when the symptoms of acute bronchitis are not treated well and in time.

4.  Bronchitis must not be taken lightly as this ailment can also lead to other severe conditions like pneumonia.

Whenever your child experiences cough or cold, rather than thinking it to be a simple phase take it seriously and consider a visit to your physician as it might get dangerous for the child leading to bronchitis!

# Understanding Bronchitis Condition - 16 Common Symptoms

Health is Wealth – this is what the wise men suggest and stands true in all regards.

Having loads of wealth and no health to enjoy and make fun in life makes no sense. Similarly to earn wealth you need proper health. Hence keeping healthy is the basic key to success.

In the lifestyle that we lead today we are surrounded with so much pollution and unwanted, unhygienic factors that it is a must to be cautious enough keep the ailments away form yourself. In short your health entirely lies in your own hands.

One of the most common ailments these days is the respiratory ailment. Asthma being the most known respiratory disease there are several others alongside that you must be aware of. One such ailment is bronchitis.

Bronchitis is a sort of a respiratory illness affecting the bronchial tree of our body. That is, in this ailment bronchi of our lungs becomes inflamed. It is a common disease among tobacco smokers & people ho are living in the areas where there are high levels of air pollution. In case you one among those affected with bronchitis, here are some points you must understand about this disease.

1. Bronchitis is of two kinds depending on the time it lasts for in the body - Acute bronchitis lasts for only 10-12 days. On the other hand, chronic bronchitis might also take 3 months to 2 years.

2. It is easier to prevent acute bronchitis because it is mainly caused due to some viral & bacterial infections.

3. Also there are some cases where this ailment comes from some fungus. The individual suffering with acute bronchitis experiences persistent cough along with mucus, shortness of breathe, feeling of fatigue, mild fever, mild chest pains, feeling of coldness, vibration inside chest while breathing, etc.

4. When acute bronchitis is caused due to virus, it is usually the same virus as that of common cold. In case of such viral infections, the doctors suggest that there is no need of any special medications. The only means of getting well is talking lots of rest and drinking loads of non caffeinated & non alcoholic beverages.

5. In case one is affected with acute bronchitis caused due to the bacterial infection, the usual antibiotic medications can treat him/her well. In such remember two things – one contact the doctor and take the anti-biotic that the expert suggests rather than taking just any medicine without prescription and two, increasing the humidity in the patients' house would really help. You can do this by placing wet towels all across the house or placing room humidifiers.

6. Generally, acute bronchitis lasts about 10-12 days only. Yet, it is closely followed and/or associated with flu and cold. So, many a times during the healing process coughing does not end and bronchi in the lungs keeps irritating. In case the coughing lasts longer than a month, the experts advise you to consult the physician immediately, before the conditions get worst. This is because, cough occurs for several other reasons as well.

7. Bronchitis happens chiefly due to infections such as viral, bacteria and very rarely due to fungus.

8. Remember you must not take any medications until & unless the doctor prescribes so else it might get dangerous for you.

9. The doctors in such cases usually get some essential lab tests done before prescribing the medications. These examinations are very important and must be taken very seriously.

Now before making any decisions, let us first understand the signs & symptoms of the bronchial diseases.

1. Bronchitis is a name given to the swelling of our bronchial tubes. This swelling leads to the bronchial mucosa's disability in getting rid of the mucus.

2.  This means the patient would have lot of cough, and face difficulty in breathing.

3.  The other symptoms include the following:

- Difficulty in breathing
- Breathlessness
- Coughing along with thick phlegm
- Pain in the throat
- Feeling tightness around the chest
- Mild fever
- Pain & swelling around the patient's eyes

4.  The other symptoms of bronchitis are as follows:

- Fatigue
- Headache
- Excessive sweating
- Nausea
- Chest pain

## Other Points

1.  The key difference between the other obstructive lung diseases and asthmatic bronchitis is that the latter is often reversible, both, with or without the treatment.

2.  Persons afflicted with asthma might experience certain symptom free episodes while interchanging acute asthmatic attacks last for a few minutes or a few days.

3.  Factors setting off the asthmatic attacks are quite similar to the asthmatic bronchitis (like dust, smoking, etc.).

4.  Common asthma is mainly triggered through the allergens. The common allergens imply ones arising due to season (that is weed pollens and grass tree), and the

persistent ones (like roaches, animal dander, dust, etc). Almost all asthmatic individuals are extremely sensitive to these triggers.

5.  The key causes of bronchitis are the bacterial infections. While asthmatic bronchitis is activated through tiny specks breaking through the safety walls created by cilia, a part of the bronchial tubes.

6.  Just like other COPDs, the asthmatic bronchitis involves congestion of our respiratory tract. The bronchial tubes actually produce mucus under all normal circumstances. This mucus then covers our lungs, trachea, and other important organs of the respiratory system. When the irritants are existent in our respiratory system, there is an overproduction of this mucus that consequently obstructs our airways. A continuous mucoid obstruction in the respiratory tract is the most common factor among the asthmatic bronchitis patients.

7.  These factors contribute towards the development of the asthmatic bronchitis, hyperactivity of bronchus and/or immunologic aberrations, the relentless childhood infections, etc.

8.  The persons suffering with asthma and/or the other grave sorts of chronic bronchitis become quite vulnerable towards asthmatic bronchitis.

9.  Ones who are afflicted with the chronic bronchitis, ultimately contract to asthmatic bronchitis owing to the long term exposure towards pollutants and/or environmental toxins & mainly cigarette smoking.

10. While the medical experts continue to research what exactly causes this disease by far the established fact is that the environmental factors lead to this ailment.

11. The general symptoms leading to asthmatic bronchitis include dyspnea (that is difficulty in breathing & shortness of breath), chest discomforts, cough, wheezing lasting for several weeks, general malaise or fatigue, weight loss, pain, usual feeling of soreness, high risk to catch infections, etc.

**How To Win Your War Against Bronchitis**

12. While the above mentioned factors are also seen in the common asthmatic patients, the persons suffering with asthmatic bronchitis also show rather profound symptoms. These are those symptoms that show higher frequencies as compared to a common asthma.

# Bronchitis And Its Infectious Nature – 16 Points To Remember

Bronchitis mans the chronic or acute soreness of our mucous membrane or the swelling in the tracheobronchial tree of our respiratory system. Tracheobronchial tree refers to the trachea or the windpipe & the bronchial tubes. This disease might be or might not be contagious, depending on some circumstances.

Initially you must understand that there are two types of bronchitis – Chronic or the long term one and acute bronchitis or the short term one.

Here are some essential medical details of the bronchial disease:

1. The solemn features of acute bronchitis are productive cough, fever, hypertrophy and/or increased mucus secreting tissues, chills, sore throat, headache, runny nose, back aches and general malaise. On the other hand, chronic bronchitis is the incapacitating ailment that is often caused by the persistent coughing along with a lot of production of phlegm and/or mucus by our glands of bronchi & trachea. In order to be called as the chronic bronchitis, the cough along with phlegm must persist continuously for nothing less than 3 months to two successive years.

2. Bronchitis both acute and chronic occur due to infections arising from bacteria, virus, and the environmental pollution (like chemical fumes, cigarette smoking, etc).

3. In order to diagnose bronchitis in a patient, the physician primarily notes down the health history of the patient. Then they make note of the signs of this disease. Further, the medical professional would auscultate and/or listen to the chest of the patient with the help of a stethoscope, to hear sounds of inflammation, wheezing in the lungs. The sounds vary largely as these could be – crackling, moist rales and wheezing.

4. Wheezing is the sign of the narrowing of your air passages. Sound produced by the hair being rubbed with one another is called crackling. Moist rales are heard when bubbling of fluid secretions in our bronchial tubes takes place.

## How To Win Your War Against Bronchitis

5.   The sputum culture is ordered by the medical experts when they observe a suspicious color and/or streaks of blood. This test helps to identify the kind of infection and the type of bacteria and/or virus present in the patients' respiratory tracts. This way they are able to plan the treatment of the patient in a better way. To collect the sputum for this test the lab personnel tell the patient to breathe deeply. Then the patient has to cough out that phlegm in to a container.  It is best done right in the morning prior to having breakfast and/or any sort of food intake. The results of this test come form the lab in about three days.

6.   In case of the chronic bronchitis patients sometimes the doctors use bronchoscopy. This is a method of collecting sputum for testing but in an advanced manner. In this method, the patient is given a local anesthesia. Then a tube is inserted in to the respiratory tract of the patient in order to collect his/her sputum.

7.   Further, the medical expert may also suggest to for a chest x-ray done followed by blood tests.

8.   With the results of these test the medical experts determine the right type of treatment for the patient and that his bronchitis is contagious or not. In case it is contagious, the medical experts there on employ the precautionary measures.

9.   Bronchitis of both the types acute as well as chronic can be contagious depending on their cause of occurrence. When bronchitis is caused due to some virus or bacteria, it becomes contagious.

10.   The commonly known viruses that make bronchitis contagious are adenovirus, influenza virus, and mycoplasma pneumoniae.

11.   Bronchitis can occur due to 2 types of influenza strains. These are - influenza A & influenza B. Both these strains are avoidable in case the patient takes an yearly doze of the influenza virus vaccine. This helps the individual become immunized against the virus.

12.   Adenovirus can be one among the 49 medium sized viruses that belong to the family of Adenoviridae. These are pathogenic (that is disease causing) for the human body. These

pathogens not only cause ailments in the human body's respiratory tract, but also become the reason for conjunctivitis, cystitis, and gastro-intestinal infections.

13.   Mycplasma pneumoniae is known for being the most contagious for young children & adults.

14.   Anti-biotics are not effective by any means when the bronchitis is caused due to the virus. The viral infections are self-limiting. These might clear out with in 14 days only if the bronchitis has not yet become complicated.

15.   In case the bronchitis is caused due to some underlying bacterial infection, the physician would most probably prescribe the anti-biotics so as to kill the bacteria & prevent it from spreading towards the neighboring organs. Usually, the patients take the anti-biotic medications just as prescribed by the doctor and readily accept the side effects.

16.   It is always possible to keep away form such contagious ailments with a simple trick – live a healthy & hygienic lifestyle. The individuals must take the adequate amount of nutrition in their diet. Take rest when you feel low, especially in the cold season. Wash your hands more often and regularly as this would prevent the spread of bacteria and viruses.  You must have very clean and hygienic surroundings to avoid bronchitis.

# <u>Bronchiolitis And Infants</u>

Parents can sacrifice all their lives for children, hen when their child is unwell how can they have a sound sleep?

When the child is persistently coughing & breathing with difficulty, you might be thinking that this no ordinary cough or cold. Well, check with your pediatrician as your baby might be suffering from Bronchiolitis.

Bronchitis commonly occurs in the adults. In this disorder the large airways in our body get inflamed. Bronchiolitis refers to the infants with their airways inflamed between their chest & the lungs. This term is coined from the word bronchioles, a part of the bronchi of the infants that is naturally smaller than that of an adult. Therefore the infections in this case are easily plugged & viruses enter very easily.

**When is your child at risk?**

1. At the age of 6 months, the baby becomes prone to develop bronchiolitis. Until the baby becomes 2 years old, this tendency is far too much.

2. The infants are rather more susceptible to this ailment during the winters and the early period of spring season.

3. The babies exposed to cigarettes & belch smokes also bare a high risk of catching up the said illness.

4. For infants, even the crowded environments cause the symptoms of bronchiolitis.

5. Male infants are at a higher risk to acquire bronchiolitis than the females.

6. During the first 6 months, the male infants that are formula-fed become more likely to acquire this ailment as compared to those who are breast-fed.

**How To Win Your War Against Bronchitis**

## What are the causes of bronchiolitis?

Respiratory Syncytial Virus or RSV is the key cause of bronchiolitis among the infants. The researchers have proved that RSV causes major ailments among young children, mostly the infants.

The other viruses that lead to bronchilitis are as follows:

## 1. Parainfluenza Virus

This sort of virus most oft brings the pediatric respiratory infections in the infants.

## 2. Mycoplasma

This sort of virus is a crucial cause of pneumonia & several other disorders linked to the respiratory system.

## 3. Adenoviruses

This virus commonly causes ailments like conjunctivitis and several others related to the respiratory system.

## 4. Influenza Virus

This sort of virus enters the human body's respiratory tract and leads to the individuals suffering with cold, cough & some extent bronchitis.

## What are the symptoms?

1. The baby begins to have a runny & stuffy nose along with meek cough. This is the key symptom of bronchiolitis among infants.

2. Next the child would suffer from varied breathing difficulties that is both in the inhaling and exhaling part.

3.  Just in a day or 2, the baby would have increased breathing difficulty along with rapid wheezing & cough. By this time, you must get aware as the heartbeats would have become very unusually fast.

4.  While all the above symptoms are a must, they are often accompanied with the others like fever and/or cooler body temperature & reduced appetite.

## How can the medical experts diagnose bronchiolitis?

In case you observe the above given symptoms in your infant, you must check with a pediatrician as soon as possible. The pediatrician would first check the baby's medical history and then assess the baby with some physical examination. Further the doctor would order for some further tests that must be taken very seriously. These tests are as follows:

1. Pulsoximeter
2. Chest x-ray

## What are the treatments recommended?

1.  The child can be temporarily relieved with the first-aid.

2.  Next you must give your child lot of non-caffeinated fluids. This would control the dehydration in the child.

3.  You can opt to make use of the humidifiers and/or saline nose drops. These would help mucus to lighten out very quickly.

4.  At times, the medical experts recommend that the parents and/or caregivers should bring their infant to a hospital so as to get them well-supervised care such as giving the fluids & oxygen as & when needed and giving the right humidified atmosphere. One very important thing in this case would be that the child would get proper medical care.

**How To Win Your War Against Bronchitis**

## Is bronchiolitis preventable?

Once your child is saved from a bronchiolitis attack, you must not risk him/her with another episode of the ailment. So, you must undertake the preventive measures that are as follows:

1. While the dicey seasons for the infant like winters and early spring season, make sure to keep your child away from persons suffering with cough, cold and flu.

2. Make sure that as a parent and/or a caregiver, you must wash your hands every time before handling the infant.

3. In case you cough or sneeze, you must use a tissue or a handkerchief to cover your mouth well enough.

4. In case you are likely to become ill, request someone to take over your responsibility for a few days.

# <u>Bronchitis - Symptoms And Treatment</u>

Bronchitis is quite a known chronic disease. Here are some interesting & basic facts about this ailment.

1.   This disease was quite common even in those days yet the developments in the medicinal field have seen now seen many alternatives to treat the said condition.

2.   The pulmonary disorders are rather common among the children. This doesn't imply that the adults are untouched with the same. As a matter of fact, living in the modern age polluted cities, amidst smokers, industries and racing cars all of us are prone to the disease.

3.   In case your bronchi are inflamed, there are chances for you to have bronchitis that is a known obstructive pulmonary disorder or illness.

4.   Bronchitis can be divided in to the acute or short term and the chronic or long term category.

5.   Bronchitis can occur in any age.

6.   It is quite closely associated with the flues and colds.

7.   In case the bronchitis is left uncured, it can lead to severe pneumonia.

8.   Bronchitis is indeed common among the smokers.

**Acute Bronchitis**

1.   Acute bronchitis' symptoms are quite similar to flu.

2.   It lasts only for a short term.

3.   Individuals suffering with the viral infections are often susceptible to the acute bronchitis.

**How To Win Your War Against Bronchitis**

4. This ailment is contagious & generally begins with dry cough that often happens at night. Within a few days, the cough would progress. Quite soon the person would suffer with other symptoms like fever, fatigue, and headache. Curing this cough might take many weeks or many months. This is because healing process in such cases is very slow, especially in your bronchial tubes.

5. In case you are suffering with cough for a month or more, your doctor could refer you to check with an ENT expert so as to ensure if there are some other causes of the irritation. Yet, if your bronchial tubes remain irritated, this can lead to the asthmatic conditions.

6. In acute bronchitis, your passage ways constrict due to infection caused by some virus or bacteria. In case the ailment is due to bacteria, the apt antibiotic regimen can do the trick to cure the ailment. It is always advised to visit the doctor to get a medical diagnosis. Remember taking any medicine with out the doctor's prescription could make the disorder rather worse.

7. Persistent cough & wheezing also imply that you might be suffering with acute bronchitis. The constricted bronchial tubes create the wheezing sound every time we breathe. While this disorder can be cleared up in a few days, in some cases it might take several months or weeks as well. Remember in such a situation, you must take lot of rest and drink lots & lots of water or juices.

8. A simple home remedy to fight back this disease is placing wet blankets & towels in varied places in the house to increase the humidity there. Room humidifiers are also a good option for such patients.

9. Smoking is anyways injurious to health but in case of the bronchial patients, it can be disastrous. So, the smokers suffering with acute bronchitis must quit the habit of smoking before the condition gets worst.

**Chronic Bronchitis**

1. This is an ongoing condition.

2.  Curing this might take several months, or even years.

3.  The environmental factors that lead to this ailment are exposure to fumes, smoke, dust, odors, etc.

4.  Chronic bronchitis is incurable, so the patients must consult their doctor well enough to identify the triggers. They should then remove as many triggers as possible form their environment in order to keep healthy.

5.  Remember, in this ailment prevention is equivalent to cure so you must work on removing the triggers else, it could be dangerous for you.

6.  Consulting the doctor, they would suggest you several laboratory tests like test for pulmonary function & blood gases in arteries, chest x-rays, and sputum culture. Generally thee test are also done for the patients of acute bronchitis.

7.  Just like acute bronchitis, smoking can make the situation worst for the patients of chronic bronchitis as well. So you must quit this bad habit in order to keep healthy and get rid of this ailment.

8.  A healthy & active lifestyle is unbeatable at the end of the day. Practicing all preventive measures can avoid bronchitis and many other ailments for all individuals.

The prime symptoms of bronchitis are:

i.      coughing
ii.     excessive mucus
iii.    fever
iv.     pain in the chest
v.      inflammation
vi.     discomfort
vii.    wheezing

These symptoms can further lead to the other respiratory problems like:

i.      sinusitis

ii.     asthma

iii.    complicated pneumonia

## Diagnose & Treatments

1. While bronchitis is a very common respiratory disorder, it is often misdiagnosed in the absence of proper para clinical & physical examinations. To get an accurate diagnose, laboratory analysis & pulmonary tests are a must.

2. Bronchitis calls for special attention before the damage is enhanced further. When the infection is bacterial, fever is the chief indication. In around 80% cases, the treatment as accomplished in just 5-10 days with the right anti-biotics. Remember, the anti-biotic or any medication must be taken with the doctor's advise else it could be devastating.

3. Antibiotics have several side effects like abdominal pain, diarrhea, rashes, etc. that can't be neglected. These cause a lot of discomfort for the patient. Yet they are acceptable only if they are absolutely necessary.

4. In case the infection is caused due to virus, or other agents, antibiotics are not effective. In such periods the only treatment is to rest for long time period, use room humidifiers, and hydrate the patients' body with lot of water and juices. In case the things do not get fine with in a few days, you must consult a doctor. It might be pneumonia and/or asthma bronchitis.

5. When the cause of bronchitis is obstructions in your bronchial tubes owing to inflammation in your respiratory tract, tissues, organs and the mucous membranes, it causes irritation and increased secretion of the mucus. Such gathering of mucus in your bronchial tubes causes difficulty in breathing, wheezing sound and coughing.

6. Bronchodilators are the medications administered to the patients who have a difficulty in breathing. These help in re-establishing the process of respiration. These are commonly prescribed to the patients suffering with chronic bronchitis & asthma.

7. Bronchitis could be dangerous and it is advisable to get treated as soon as possible to avoid all complications!

## <u>Curing Bronchitis – 0ver 25 Points To Remember</u>

Bronchitis is a respiratory disease very commonly found now a days. In this condition the air passages in our lungs are inflamed. This disease can either be chronic, acute, or asthmatic.

Acute bronchitis is short term. Caused by the viral infection beginning in the sinuses and/or the nose spreading in to the air passages, it is believed to be cured generally in 10-12 days.

The chronic bronchitis occurs when cough in the sputum stays for three months and up to a year. This is the rather dangerous disease that occurs mainly among the smokers. It is also known as COPD that is chronic obstructive pulmonary disease. Once diagnosed in the early stage it is curable.

The symptoms though somewhat similar in both the cases vary at some point. The signs & symptoms of acute bronchitis are:

i.        Wheezing

ii.       Fever

iii.      Fatigue

iv.      Sore throat

v.        Cough producing mucus

vi.      Burning sensation in the chest

The symptoms of chronic bronchitis enlist:

i.        Wheezing

ii.       Chronic cough yielding excessive mucus

iii.      Inability to breath

iv.      Blue-tinged lips

v.        Swelling of ankle, feet, leg, etc.

Some other facts about bronchitis are as follows:

1.  Viral infection causes acute bronchitis and bacteria.

## How To Win Your War Against Bronchitis

2. Usually, acute bronchitis is transmitted from one patient to another.

3. Chronic bronchitis is often caused due to cigarette smoking & long-term exposure with irritants such as dust, grain and air pollution.

4. When you go far an examination, the doctor listens to the chest and the back, examining the throat.  He then draws some blood & takes that for culturing the lung secretions in the check ups. In case the doctor suspects COPD or pneumonia, he would also make you undergo a chest x-ray.

5. The simple means of preventing these ailments are –

  i.  Keeping away from the irritants & air pollutants.

  ii.  Taking yearly flu & pneumococcal vaccination to avoid infections leading to the chronic bronchitis exacerbation and/or acute bronchitis.

The treatments involved in the cases of these ailments are as follows:

1. Usually viruses get cleared with in 7-10 days in the cases of acute bronchitis.

2. For this the doctors recommend the cough medications including expectorants.

3. They also suggest you to place room humidifiers in your house.

4. You are always advised to drink loads of fluids such as water and juices to get rid of the growing symptoms.

5. In case it is an infection cause due to virus or bacteria, it is a must to check with the doctor first.

6. Usually the doctors prescribe antibiotics.

7. In some cases the doctors prescribe bronchodilators, such as Albuterol. This medication helps an easy opening of the airways in our bronchi. They also effect the corticosteroids that is inhaled or taken in orally so as to reduce the inflammation & mucus.

8. Leading a healthy and hygienic lifestyle is a must. Quit smoking and make use of air conditioners, air filters and curtains in the house in order to breathe clean air in the house. Changing your lifestyle is also a helpful remedy. You need to stop smoking.

9. Plant a steam or humidifier in house, especially bathroom.

10. Get used to having lots of liquids such as water and juices.

11. While the infection is active, you must take rest.

12. In cases of chronic bronchitis when the oxygen in the body gets low, take oxygen therapy at your home itself.

13. Focus on the dietary & nutrition supplements. Experiment with some food materials and see if they are helping to deteriorate or control the bronchial symptoms.

14. Record all the disturbances that you feel and make sure to report them to your doctor.

15. Lessen the dairy products as much as possible as they produce lot of mucus that is not good for your health while in a bronchial condition. Avoid eggs, milk, preservatives, nuts, food coloring, additives, etc.

16. Put lots of garlic & onions in the food as it is advisable in such condition.

17. The studies reveal that NAC that is N-Acetyl-Cysteine is helpful in dissolving the mucus and improving the symptoms pertaining to chronic bronchitis.

18. Zinc supplementation enhances the activities in the immune system. It protects the individual from bronchial infections and colds.

**How To Win Your War Against Bronchitis**

19. The other advisable supplements are vitamin C, quercetin, bromalein, and lactobacillus. All these supplements prevent the individual from getting afflicted with the infections & relieve him/her from the bronchitis symptoms.

20. Usage of herbs to treat varied ailments is a very old & successful concept. Yet this also has its advantages and disadvantages. The herbs can land up in side effects if not taken with proper prescription and knowledge. Especially their interactions with the other supplements, medications, and other herbs.

21. Some of the well known herbs are as follows:

i. Berberis vulgaris or barberry improves the immune system functions & fights infections.

ii. Eucalyptus also known as eucalyptus globules are apt for treating the common colds & coughs. The oil made of eucalyptus helps loosening the phlegm.

iii. Mentha x piperita or peppermint is effective in place of decongestants. This contains menthol that helps in thinning the mucus just like an expectorant. Peppermint also provides a calming & soothing effect for the dry coughs & sore throats.

iv. Slippery elm, also known as the ulmus fulva is known above as it is recognized by U.S. FDA (that is Food & Drug Authority) for its effectiveness & no side effects in the respiratory symptoms & sore throat.

v. Urtica dioica or Stinging nettle acts as another expectorant with anti-viral properties.

vi. Homeopathy along with standard medical attention proves indeed helpful. This is because a person's psychological, physical, and emotional all make-ups are taken in to consideration in this procedure.

# <u>An Overview Of Bronchitis - 30 Points To Understand</u>

Bronchitis is quite a known chronic disease. Here are some interesting & basic facts about this ailment.

- Charles Bedham in 1808 described this disease and called it bronchitis.

- This disease was quite common even in those days yet the developments in the medicinal field have seen now seen many alternatives to treat the said condition.

- The pulmonary disorders are rather common among the children. This doesn't imply that the adults are untouched with the same. As a matter of fact, living in the modern age polluted cities, amidst smokers, industries and racing cars all of us are prone to the disease.

- In case your bronchi are inflamed, there are chances for you to have bronchitis that is a known obstructive pulmonary disorder or illness.

- Bronchitis can be divided in to the acute or short term and the chronic or long term category.

- But how does one come to know that he/she is suffering with bronchitis? For this you must understand the symptoms of this disorder. These are as follows:

i. Expectorating cough
ii. Dyspnea
iii. Fatigue and/or Malaise
iv. Mild fever & chest pains
v. Coldness
vi. Vibrating chest

- Bronchitis can happen in all ages.

- The individuals who suffer with frequent flu & colds often tend to suffer with this condition.

## How To Win Your War Against Bronchitis

- In case your immune system is not strong enough, you stand a greater risk of suffering with the major complications such as chronic & asthmatic bronchitis. Also there are chances for pneumonia to settle down in your body quite easily.

- Bronchitis can be acute or chronic – in order to give the right diagnose and treat the disease well enough, your pulmonary specialist needs to be very detailed in his diagnosis. This would help him understand the disease and ailment better.

- It is a must for the responsible individual to be aware of the signs & symptoms, so as to judge your acquaintance or family member is exhibiting the bronchitis symptoms. Knowing the symptoms well would help you identify the patient easily and hence seek medical help in time.

- Like all other ailment, even for bronchitis, it is the best to get treated at an early stage that is when the disease is yet controllable & less problematic.

## Acute Bronchitis

- Acute bronchitis' symptoms are quite similar to flu.

- It lasts only for a short term.

- Individuals suffering with the viral infections are often susceptible to the acute bronchitis.

- This ailment is contagious & generally begins with dry cough that often happens at night. Within a few days, the cough would progress. Quite soon the person would suffer with other symptoms like fever, fatigue, and headache. Curing this cough might take many weeks or many months.  This is because healing process in such cases is very slow, especially in your bronchial tubes.

- In case you are suffering with cough for a month or more, your doctor could refer you to check with an ENT expert so as to ensure if there are some other causes of the irritation. Yet, if your bronchial tubes remain irritated, this can lead to the asthmatic conditions.

## How To Win Your War Against Bronchitis

- In acute bronchitis, your passage ways constrict due to infection caused by some virus or bacteria. In case the ailment is due to bacteria, the apt antibiotic regimen can do the trick to cure the ailment. It is always advised to visit the doctor to get a medical diagnosis. Remember taking any medicine with out the doctor's prescription could make the disorder rather worse.

- Persistent cough & wheezing also imply that you might be suffering with acute bronchitis. The constricted bronchial tubes create the wheezing sound every time we breathe. While this disorder can be cleared up in a few days, in some cases it might take several months or weeks as well. Remember in such a situation, you must take lot of rest and drink lots & lots of water or juices.

- A simple home remedy to fight back this disease is placing wet blankets & towels in varied places in the house to increase the humidity there. Room humidifiers are also a good option for such patients.

- Smoking is anyways injurious to health but in case of the bronchial patients, it can be disastrous. So, the smokers suffering with acute bronchitis must quit the habit of smoking before the condition gets worst.

**Chronic Bronchitis**

- This is an ongoing condition.

- Curing this might take several months, or even years.

- The environmental factors that lead to this ailment are exposure to fumes, smoke, dust, odors, etc.

- Chronic bronchitis is incurable, so the patients must consult their doctor well enough to identify the triggers. They should then remove as many triggers as possible form their environment in order to keep healthy.

**How To Win Your War Against Bronchitis**

- Remember, in this ailment prevention is equivalent to cure so you must work on removing the triggers else, it could be dangerous for you.

- Consulting the doctor, they would suggest you several laboratory tests like test for pulmonary function & blood gases in arteries, chest x-rays, and sputum culture. Generally thee test are also done for the patients of acute bronchitis.

- Just like acute bronchitis, smoking can make the situation worst for the patients of chronic bronchitis as well. So you must quit this bad habit in order to keep healthy and get rid of this ailment.

- A healthy & active lifestyle is unbeatable at the end of the day. Practicing all preventive measures can avoid bronchitis and many other ailments for all individuals.

How To Win Your War Against Bronchitis


This Product Is Brought To You By

# DAVID A OSEI